Taste Life!

The Organic Choice

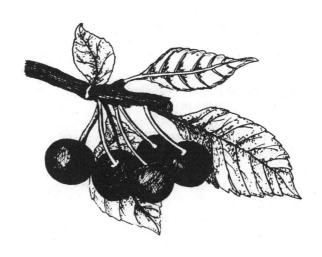

Taste Life! The Organic Choice
Edited by David Richard and Dorie Byers

Copyright ©1998 Vital Health Publishing

Printed in the United States of America by United Graphics, Inc., Mattoon, IL on recycled paper using soy based ink.

Cover and Text Design by Studio 2D, Champaign, IL.

Cover photograph by Stan Jorstad.

Illustrations by Susan Cavaciuti.

Vital Health Publishing
P.O. Box 544
Bloomingdale, IL 60108

ISBN: 1-890612-08-1

Acknowledgments

The joy of a project like this one is that it is so much larger than any one or two individuals. If we traced the history of the organic movement to its deepest roots, there would not be room in all of these pages to list those who have helped to make this book possible. Notwithstanding, there are a number of individuals whose assistance has been instrumental in bringing the perspectives of Taste Life! together.

We are grateful to Dr. Don Gray of the Canberra Organic Grower's Association for his contribution of Lady Eve Balfour's speech and for the gift of his time in our correspondence. Lisa Bell has similarly helped us with Gene Kahn's chapter which Cascadian Farms has generously donated. We sincerely appreciate the permission granted by Susan Davies and Michael Dobson of the Anthroposophic Press for the Koepf chapter on Biodynamic Agriculture. We are also grateful to Professor Combs and his associates at Cornell University for allowing us to reprint their article.

The trade association and certifying agencies of the organic community have been both kind and helpful, particularly Holly Givens of The Organic Trade Association (OTA), Fred Kirschenman of Farm Verified Organic (FVO) and Marc Schwartz of the Organic Growers and Buyers Association (OGBA).

Trish Crapo would like to thank the following individuals in helping her compile material for the sidebar to her essay: Linda Lutz at the Organic Trade Association, Kathy Ruhf at the New England Small Farm Institute, and Cathy Greene and Howard Baker at the USDA.

Anthony Rodale and Pat Flexer of Rodale Publication were helpful to us, respectively, in contacting Bargyla Rateaver and in compiling the Rodale materials.

We thank Stan and Steve Jorstad for digging through stacks and drawers of color negatives to locate a cover photograph for this book—

just at the time when Stan's photo-journal of our national parks, *These Rare Lands*, was being released.

We enjoyed reading all of the essays submitted for our Taste Life! essay contest and trust that the book will be worth the wait for those who won a copy.

Ian Diamond of The Organic Connection deserves our special thanks for his reading of the manuscript and helpful suggestions.

Our ongoing thanks to Denise Huisman who compiled the numerous drafts of the manuscript and to Gretchen Weishuber who laid out both the cover and text for the book.

Finally, we are grateful to Elwood Richard (David's dad) of The Fruitful Yield Corp. and Now Foods for his support and encouragement throughout this project.

It has been a blessing to prepare the "meal" of this book together. Hopefully, the aromas and flavors of the different essays spread out on the table together will encourage people to accept our invitation to join the organic banquet. It is truly a feast for all!

Contents

Foreword

When the idea for this book first came to me, the image of a crusade arose involving a titanic struggle between two systems of agriculture: an organic system (the forces of "good") and an industrialized system (the forces of "evil"). Underlying these two systems, in my mind at least, were the ideologies of the naturalist and the technologist.

As *Taste Life!* has gradually taken form, this image has come to be replaced by one which is less apocalyptic and more humane. I now consider the patience of the earth itself, perhaps somewhat wearied and worn by the foolishness of our inventions, yet nevertheless forbearing and willing to restore in the abundance of its fertility and in the regeneration of its cycles and seasons. I also think of all of those people who are literally starving due to lack of proper nourishment or who are suffering, in varying degrees of toxemia, from eating unhealthy food. This book is written both for the patient, forbearing earth and for its hungry, suffering inhabitants. While it can neither literally restore the earth nor provide real nourishment for its inhabitants, it can help to restore a sense of trust and gratitude toward the earth and to nourish the thoughts and decisions of its inhabitants.

Taste Life! is about a philosophy of life, therefor, which will either stand or fall on its own merits. I am encouraged that so many people are now willing to consider this philosophy for themselves and their families. I am certain that Sir McCarrison, Sir Howard, Prof. Steiner, Lady Balfour, J.I. Rodale and Prof. Albrecht, along with the many other pioneers of the organic movement, would also be pleased with this trend.

I encourage you to *Taste Life!* through the essays in this book. Yet what you taste and how you taste it, in terms of the "food on your plate," remain as personal decisions for you to consider.

DAVID RICHARD

The health of the people
is really the foundation
upon which all their happiness
and all their powers as a state depend.

—BENJAMIN DISRAELI

Gaea or Ge, the personification of the Earth,
called Tellus by the Romans;
described as the first being that sprang from chaos.

—BULLFINCH'S MYTHOLOGY

How many prayers have been raised
in thanksgiving for the fruits of the earth?
Nourishment kindles the fire of gratitude.

—EDITOR

Introduction

Ever since he was old enough to walk, our son has picked fresh produce from the garden and enjoyed eating it on the spot. Green beans, sugar snap peas, cherry tomatoes, sweet corn, and radishes would be included in his harvest. After a quick brushing off, he would enjoy them where he stood, still warm from the sun and fresh from the vine. Having heard from many parents of the struggle to have their children eat vegetables, I counted my blessings on how easy this was.

So, you ask, what does my child's eating habits have to do with this book? The answer is that I garden organically. Since the food is grown without pesticides, herbicides, or synthetic fertilizers, I have no concerns about my child's potential exposure to these chemicals from his garden meals and snacks. I have complete confidence that he can pick food from the garden and eat it where he stands. The organic crops that we raise give my family a healthy wholesome supply of produce.

I first became aware of the importance of organic food when I was a young adult and read Rachel Carson's book *Silent Spring*. It had a profound effect on how I looked at the earth and changed the way I treated it. At the time, I was far removed from gardens and growing foods. I had moved away from the farm where I grew up and was making my way in a large city. Several years later I married and found myself living on some acreage that had been overgrazed by horses and left in less than optimal shape. My husband and I made a vow to take care of the land and leave it in better shape than we found it. Land stewardship became a part of our lives and I found my evenings full of reading about organics and the care of the land. My days were filled with putting the readings into practice. A decade later, I find that these practices have given me a more mature commitment to organic food production and consumption that was only in its infancy when I read Rachel Carson's words years before.

From this commitment came the opportunity to help compile this book. This process has reaffirmed many of my beliefs as well as adding to them. I encourage you to read the essays contained in this book in the hope that you will find the knowledge to support and enjoy organic foods.

There are many voices in the organic foods movement. They come from the past and present. Many of the voices from the past ring as true now as they did when their ideas were originally spoken. Besides echoing the voices of the past, present day voices often add more ideas and insights to the organic movement. These essays have made me realize that there is so much more to organic foods than growing and eating them.

Read the excerpt from one of Robert Rodale's books. He, along with his father J.I., present a message that encourages the adoption of organic practices. It is a message that is comfortingly familiar to those of us who garden organically, for their years of experience in pioneering the organic movement in this country have inspired and encouraged us. Many people who work the land organically have turned to these words, and still turn to them for the practical information and the words of inspiration that they contain.

This book includes insights from many other individauls in the organic movement in this country. Travel to the field with Frank Ford and listen as he recalls the years he farmed organically and formed his business. Take an intimate trip through the soil with organic pioneer Barglya Rateaver. Fred Kirschenmann is another organic farmer who offers information about feeding the world population with organic foods.

The turn of the century brought us a few people who looked at the soil and growing crops in a unique way, lending their voices to the beginnings of organic gardening and farming. These were voices that understood the soil and how important the care of it was and is for quality food production. Learn from Sir Albert Howard, who worked in India to improve the spent soil there. Lady Eve Balfour, whose farm was the site of an ecologically designed agricultural research project, explains to us that soil and its care became the key for organically produced food.

Some of the voices are unique in their outlook. Excerpts of the Biodynamic approach to organic gardening will give you an insight into ideas taught by the philosopher-scientist Dr. Rudolf Steiner and his followers. Another unique view is from farmer-photographer Michael Ableman's excerpts about native farmers' relationships to the earth.

The observations he makes from his travels will give you a feel for the stewardship of land in other countries where small farmers tend crops in traditional ways to keep food on their tables. Catch a glimpse of the culinary delights enjoyed by cooking with organic produce as narrated by organic cookbook author Leslie Cerier.

The history, business, and practice involved in the growing of organic foods is covered by Gene Kahn of Cascadian Farms, who gives a great overview of organic food production with other aspects of organics covered. Marc Schwartz gives insight into the marketing and development of organic foods products in a travel monologue through the recent history of the organic movement from the driver's seat of a VW van.

Britt Bailey and Marc Lappe contribute a collective voice that lends credence to gardening and farming organically to avoid the use of potentially harmful chemicals. This issue is additionally brought close to home by Dana Pratt, a mother and organic gardener who has the primary concern of her family at the forefront of organic food consumption.

Overall, the message given by these and other voices that are included in the book are positive in nature. There is a tone of hopefulness for the future of organic foods and a long term view of providing and consuming healthful foods that are grown without exposure to potentially harmful substances. This hopefulness can be heard even in the words written some time ago by the pioneers of the organic movement. The idea of growing more healthful food was started many decades ago by those whose names are familiar to us but who are no longer with us and was picked up by a second generation of pioneers whose names we are just getting to know. The ongoing result is an improvement in the quality of life for those who make the organic choice.

I invite you to open the pages of this book and read with the intention of learning about organic foods and why consuming them can help you to improve your quality of life. It can be informative and frequently inspiring reading. Some of the essays will be like taking a walk through the fields with the gardeners and farmers. Others are thought provoking from the standpoint of science, philosophy, or traditional wisdom. All are well worth your time to read. With these things in mind, I invite you to enter "Taste Life! The Organic Choice."

DORIE BYERS

Organic agriculture is an ecological production management system that promotes and enhances biodiversity, biological cycles and soil biological activity. It is based on minimal use of off-farm inputs and on management practices that restore, maintain and enhance ecological harmony. "Organic" is a labeling term that denotes products produced under the authority of the Organic Foods Production Act. The principal guidelines for organic production are to use materials and practices that enhance the ecological balance of natural systems and that integrate the parts of the farming system into an ecological whole. Organic agriculture practices cannot ensure that products are completely free of residues; however, methods are used to minimize pollution from air, soil and water. Organic food handlers, processors and retailers adhere to standards that maintain the integrity of organic agricultural products. The primary goal of organic agriculture is to optimize the health and productivity of interdependent communities of soil, life, plants, animals and people.

NATIONAL ORGANIC STANDARDS BOARD, 1995

The answer to health
will be found in the soil
to a great extent.

—J.I. RODALE

Organic food has superior nutritional quality
as a result of its growth on fertile soil.

—ROBERT RODALE

Organically grown food almost always has
a recognizable good old-fashioned taste.

—RODALE PRESS EDITORS

What's It All About?

ROBERT RODALE

EXCERPTED FROM *THE BASIC BOOK OF ORGANICALLY GROWN FOODS* BY PERMISSION OF THE EDITORS OR ORGANIC GARDENING AND FARMING, RODALE PRESS, EMMAUS, PA 1972.

"Organic food" is grown in soil rich in organic matter. Organic matter—or humus—is the living part of the soil. In that moist, woodsy part of the soil, exist the unaccountable billions of bacteria, fungi and other minute organisms which give soil remarkable powers to feed tremendous amounts of minerals, and other nutrients to plant roots.

The past 150 years of large-scale farming have depleted soil organic matter. Now, many soils contain less than 1 per cent humus. Manure is spread on fields less often, and the stalks or other waste portions of plants are often removed from the land. Many soils are therefore less alive than they used to be, and the crops they produce are less healthy and sometimes are lower in nutritional value.

Organically grown food varies in quality according to the area in which it is grown, but almost always it has a recognizable good, old-fashioned taste which is sadly lacking in supermarket food. An organically raised chicken, for example, is fed no drugs to stimulate growth and is allowed to scratch in the ground and eat the worms, bugs and the other critters that are delicacies to a chicken. As a result, the meat of the bird has a hearty flavor. A member of the older generation fed an organic chicken will suddenly remember how white meat used to taste.

The word organic is crucial to the appreciation of the concept of ecological purity in food. Organically grown is a label that is easily understood by city people, who after all, know very little about farming. Organically grown means food as it used to be grown, without the latest chemical aids that have backfired on the environment in so many ways. Organically grown means food that helps the land and the bodies of people, instead of tearing them down. Organic is power to people who were just manipulated into thinking that food like fat, drugged beef is "quality."

The enemies of organic farming realize, to their great disgust, the tremendous value of the word organic. They see how it has caused food consumers to wonder about all that chemical junk they are eating. Even more important, the chemical proponents sense in the popularity of the word organic the seeds of a genuine revolution, which will eventually deprive them of their markets for food additives and chemical fertilizers. The chemical salesmen know the word organic is telling the public that the ordinary food they eat is not quite as natural or as pure as it could be.

People are becoming increasingly aware of the benefits or organic foods...The lack of chemical residues ranks as the number one benefit because it is the one people think of first. It is the advantage that convinces most to start eating organically grown food.

Humus-rich soil improves the food value of plants to providing them with all the nutrients they need in the proper balance. Balance is the key word. When artificial fertilizers are used, the plants' roots are often saturated with an abundance of one nutrient, making it difficult for them to pick up others they need just as much. Since artificial fertilizers present their food in soluble form, the plant can't be selective and you can almost say it is forced to use whatever is given to it.

Organic food is not debased by unnecessary processing. You can't call a loaf of white bread organic even if it is made from organically grown wheat. Having taken the life from the grain, you have eliminated its right to bear the label "organic." Fortunately, most growers and suppliers of organic foods appreciate that users want a product natural in all respects, and they strive to treat their food naturally. And when you grow your own organic food you have control over it every step of the way. Most important, the average organic gardener doesn't have the knowledge or the means to over-process food. It usually takes a lot of skill and expensive equipment.

When you buy tomatoes in the store, you are getting the fruit of a plant that meets the farmer's requirements but not necessarily yours. The same could be said of almost every fruit, vegetable or grain. When a farmer grows tomatoes, for example, he wants plants whose fruit will ripen in unison, be easy to pick, stand up under shipment and yield the maximum number of bushels or tons per acre. Your wishes as a consumer are observed only so long as they don't conflict with his production problems. But when you grow tomatoes in your own garden, you can pick the variety that fully meets your needs. If you want high vitamin C content, you can grow DOUBLERICH of HIGH-C tomatoes. If you want plenty of vitamin A you can select CARO-RED. The day may come when supermarkets will handle superior varieties of plants because their customers are demanding them.

Commercial farmers today are too concerned with events of today and are making excuses for the failures they are breeding for tomorrow. They know organic matter is essential to the health of the soil, and they know their farming methods are draining the organic matter away little by little each year. But they have to pay off loans on their big new machines, so they use methods they know are unsound to get highest yields. Tomorrow is time enough to put back the humus, they figure.

Even though the farmer is the custodian of the soil, you can't blame him entirely for slowly wearing it out. In our modern agricultural establishment, there are hordes of people who are helping with that job. The chemical companies are spending millions of dollars to get new pesticides cleared for farm use, but they spend practically nothing to find out what the pesticide residues are doing as they accumulate in the soil. About a third of all the research done by the state experiment stations is directly financed by companies with some product to sell to the farmer. Many new farm scientists graduating each year have had their educations paid for by chemical company scholarships and grants.

Sir Albert Howard, an English agricultural advisor to the Indian state of Indore, first thought out the concept of growing plants, and husbanding animals without using synthetic chemicals. Partly, his development of natural gardening and farming was a reaction to necessity. The area of India where he worked was so poor that local farmers couldn't afford to buy fertilizers imported from other areas. So Sir Albert had to devise ways to recycle the natural nutrients available locally— the manure of animals and the waste plant materials that would otherwise be burned or ignored.

J.I. Rodale first read about Sir Albert Howard's ideas in the late 1930's. Even then, the United States was so industrialized and technologically "advanced" that it was possible to see that what Sir Albert was predicting could easily happen. The American Dust Bowl experience of the Depression years was graphic evidence of the disruption of the cycle of life. But there were signs of trouble everywhere. Food quality was low. Pollution was intruding on our lives. Disease caused by physical degeneration-not just by microbes-was increasing. J.I. Rodale noted with dismay that the grim harvest predicted by Sir Albert and other philosophers of the conservation school was about to be reaped.

J.I. first used the word "organic" to describe the natural method of gardening and farming, mainly because compost, humus and the organic fraction of the soil were emphasized so strongly. However, even in 1942, when *Organic Gardening and Farming* was born, J.R. Rodale saw that this method was more than just a way to husband the soil and grow plants and animals. He proclaimed that to be "organic" was to know and to understand the lessons of nature in all ways, and to use that knowledge to evaluate all of the blessings of science and technology. What good was it, he said, to grow food without using chemical fertilizers or pesticides, and then to process that food so that its content of vitamins and minerals would de depleted seriously? In fact, not caring whether he was called an extremist or a crackpot, J.I. Rodale created what might now be called a "strict constructionist" interpretation of natural life under the banner of organiculture. If it is synthetic, avoid it, he said. If it goes through a factory, examine it with special care. Follow the dictates of the cycle of life when growing things, he advised, and you will be blessed with foods of surpassing taste and quality that are less troubled by insects or disease.

There is only one way to make America more natural, more reasonable in its burden on the ecosphere. That is the organic method. If everyone became organic-minded and backed it up with organic actions, the dire predictions for America's future could surely be thwarted. In an organic America, the sales of chemical pollutants would end. There would be no problem with additives in food and no DDT to worry about. Garbage would be less of a problem because almost everyone would be sure that organic wastes were being composted. Sewage would enrich farm fields instead of polluting rivers, lakes and harbors. Automobile smog would be minimized because more people would be living on small homesteads, raising much of their own food instead of commuting into large cities to work. Pollution would be virtually eliminated in an organic world.

Can you accept that? Or do you think we're going too far in saying that a method of gardening and farming can save the world? Well, the organic method is more than just a way to garden and farm. It is a natural philosophy of living, outlining a way for people to complete the cycle of resource use which is now broken completely in almost every city and town in this country. When you are organic you use the energy of the sun and the fertility of the soil to produce food and even clothing for your family, without expecting the aid of powerful chemicals which cause pollution. Far more important, however, an organic person puts what is used back into the resource bank upon which future generations will depend. When garbage and sewage and crop wastes are returned to the soil, we are making life a complete cycle instead of a drain down which the world's accumulated resources are flushed.

We organic people thus hold in our hands the key to the survival of America as a workable sensible place to live. No one can overestimate today the importance of the organic method to human survival. Suddenly, the organic movement is growing faster than ever.

Already you see the word "organic" cropping up more and more frequently in the writings of people who are truly ahead of their time. Many years ago, Frank Lloyd Wright planned an important seed with his ideas of organic architecture. He thought buildings should blend with and reflect the true nature of their sites. At least in a symbolic way that concept foretold the closing of the broken link of the cycle of life, which is the essence of the organic method of growing plants and animals.

As appealing as these high-type organic ideas are, they provide little place for the average person to grab on—no handle on which individual people can exert leverage. But we can all bury our garbage in the earth. We can all pick the bugs off our potato plants, instead of using poison sprays. And we can grow much of our own food—and food of the finest, purest quality—instead of using the plastic food sold in supermarkets. The organic method of gardening and farming is therefore a place to start, which is what we desperately need. I firmly believe that the organic way of living points down the right road, even though that road might have a few bumps and some hills to climb. Let's hope that everyone will start understanding the world as organic people have been understanding it for 30 years.

We cannot go on forever treating the soil as a chemical laboratory
    and expect to turn out *natural food*.
What we are getting is more chemical food.
Instead of eating live matter which can readily be absorbed
    by the body,
we are consuming food which is rapidly becoming more artificial.

———————————

I believe a whole new era of agricultural research
is in the making—one that will benefit the country at large
far more than all the research of the past has done,
one that will more nearly help to create a healthy society
and keep it in close touch with the land
from which it gets its strength and sweetness . . .

———————————

Where any one item in Nature's cycle is disturbed
it will be found that others are automatically affected.
Nature consists of a chain of interrelated
    and interlocked life cycles.
Remove any one factor and you will find
that she cannot do her work effectively.

———————————

Compost is the core,
the essential foundation
of natural gardening and farming.
It is the *heart*
of the organic concept.

—JI RODALE (ALL QUOTATIONS)

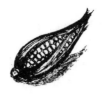

Traditional Methods of Organic Farming

MICHAEL ABLEMAN

EXCERPTS FROM *FROM THE GOOD EARTH* THOMAS AND HUDSON, LONDON, 1993; BY PERMISSION OF MR. ABLEMAN.

Introduction

My life as a farmer has always been interrupted by a photographer's wanderlust. In 1984 I left the farm to travel in the Himalaya Mountains in Nepal. But on the way there, during a stopover in Hong Kong, a friend encouraged me to take a short side trip into mainland China. This detour provided an experience that would alter the course of my life.

I had been in China for only a few days when my curiosity forced me to ignore the restrictions that kept most foreign tourists out of the countryside. I walked for several hours away from the city of Chengdu, the capital of Szechwan province, eventually up a trail to the edge of a small settlement.

I stood balancing on a narrow pathway separating the fields. All around, as far as I could see, was a network of intensive raised beds, every inch meticulously planted with a diversity of vegetables, surrounded by an elaborate network of waterways and paths. Four thousand years of Chinese agriculture seemed to merge in this moment. I stood in awe of a system so sound that the same fields could be farmed over and over for forty centuries without any apparent depletion of soil or loss of fertility.

I found myself photographing like crazy. I had so often struggled to reconcile my farmer's hand and photographer's eye. Now in China the two aspects inside me came together.

Over the next six years I traveled to many countries seeking out the remote, often-neglected traditional farmers. I wanted to understand how my own approach to food and farming—as a natural bond between community and a generous earth—had been lived out for thousands of years, how and why our society has destroyed that bond, and how we can redeem it.

I later returned to China to study the oldest agricultural tradition in the world. In Africa I visited ancient Kenyan farming cultures, and in the mountains of Burundi I saw a remarkable interconnection between farmer and farm. In the fields of Sicily, where rocks seem to outnumber crops, I stayed with farmers who still maintain the traditions that once fed much of Europe. In the Andes I witnessed a culture's incredible adaptation to a vertical terrain, and I was repeatedly drawn back to the land of the Hopi, to a people who have survived in a harsh desert ecology solely through their deeper understanding and connection to the earth and its spiritual forces.

Exploring food sources also took me to the landscapes of modern industrial farms where earth-crunching machinery and deadly chemical sprays at times suggested scenes from a war-ravaged nightmare. This was the provocative contrast.

But my wanderings did not stop there. This alone would have only offered a vision of what we have lost.

I wanted to discover some examples of hope. I began recording those who have quietly been working to restore the earth garden—to bring back purity, nourishment, taste, and beauty to our food. Here on these farms and gardens of the future a growing number of visionaries have combined ancient wisdom, new and often unorthodox science, and a lively sense of aesthetics to create living farms that produce living food. From the fields and orchards of organic farms, to urban ghettos where food gardens have been built on abandoned lots, to communities where developmentally disabled people are nurtured through working with the land, small steps are being taken—small, but powerful, steps.

I traveled over 100,000 miles and across five continents. Through my travels came the realization that a common thread connects all these stewards of the earth. Titus, the Hopi farmer singing to his corn on a remote desert mesa in Arizona; a community of some sixty people in the steep mountains of Peru, working together to plant a field of potatoes for those who cannot work; Dick Harter, an organic rice grower in Chico, California, who cares as much about the number of birds on his farm as the number of grains of rice; and Alta Felton, an eighty-year old woman whose cotton, black-eyed peas, and yams grow below the railroad tracks in South Philadelphia—all represent a small but far-reaching movement: they all reclaim and renew the earth one spadeful at a time, one bucket of compost at a time, one handful of seeds at a time.

Colquepata, Peru

As the truck forged deep into the mountains, glimpses of life began to draw me in. A dense mist filled a canyon, concealing all but the most distant views. As the sun burned through, the vertical face of a mountain came clear, broken into hundreds of mysterious shapes of brown and green: terraced fields of potatoes, barley, and beans.

Made by hand and expertly engineered by eye, some terraces were no longer than a suburban front lawn yet contained more than thirty varieties of potatoes. In fact, some terraces, as I later learned, had been in continuous use since the time of the Incas, whose short, hundred-year reign had created a range of tools and techniques that allowed people to flourish in a difficult environment. I imagined the many hands and ancient footplows that had made their indelible mark on that steep hillside—a land worked for centuries—yet I could see virtually no erosion.

Southern Yunnan, China

Our host was a quiet farmer named Jiang. Over the course of my visit we shared thoughts about growing and the earth. Philosophical discussion was often difficult as my friends struggled to interpret the local dialect. But in the fields, farmer to farmer, Jiang and I could often understand each other without too many words. I began to get an intuitive sense of how well adapted this farming was as I came to see the complex techniques that had evolved over centuries of trial and error.

Here was an integrated system far more sophisticated than my own and much of what I had seen in the West. On permanent raised garden beds, ten harvests of different crops could occur in one year. All required only minimal space, water, and external inputs, yet produced sustained high yields. Soil fertility was maintained year after year through composting and through rotating food crops with "green manure" crops (grown specifically to be turned under, adding natural nitrogen and organic matter to the soil). Some beds were surrounded by waterways supporting other nitrogen-fixing plants—food for ducks and geese and food for the soil. All resources and waste materials were carefully managed, with everything used, reused, and then used again.

Refined craft and a commitment to sustaining their soils had been passed down through generations. While the broader Chinese environment has been devastated by political and economic pressures, the "simple peasants" in their fields retain a knowledge that has enabled them to bring forth food on the same land year after year, century after century—an accomplishment unheard-of in the West.

Hopiland, Arizona

I had come to drive my friend to his field. This outing was not to work—his body was no longer able—but only to look and talk.

We drove to the top of a rock outcropping that rose from his land. From here we could see the whole of his field and beyond, into millions of acres of open desert. There was nothing more sacred, nothing more important in this man's life than his field of corn. I could see it the moment we arrived from the way he touched his plants and looked down and beyond the rows.

Burundi, Africa

The first time I saw a *rugo* I was amazed. This cluster of round thatched homes looked as if it had been seeded and had grown right out of the landscape. Each one was surrounded with concentric circles of terraced cropland planted with grains and vegetables, hedged with grasses for feed and to control erosion.

Each *rugo* provided for several generations of a family, their animals, and their food, there was even a separate hut for compost.

Over the weeks of spring planting, as I watched the women tend their fields, barefoot and consumed in the rhythmic dance of hoe and seed, I observed true integration—a way of life a child learns riding on its mother's back as she works, a closed circle where homes are ringed with crops and humans and animals feed each other and the earth.

Overview

Half of our world neighbors are supported by subsistence farming and live quietly off the land. We seldom hear much about them unless there is a major famine, civil war, or natural disaster.

They are silent, for the rhythm of their lives requires little from the outside. Yet the communities they live in and the way in which they have sustained themselves has much to offer our modern world where we no longer understand the most basic skill of feeding ourselves and the land.

It is not out of nostalgia or blind romance that we must listen to these cultures. There is nothing romantic about their day-to-day lives. The experience of Chinese farmers working in harmony with their families and the land does not dispel the horrors of Tiananmen Square: in the Peruvian village where I stayed, a family committed suicide by drinking the Western-made pesticides that were supposed to bring them a better harvest. Tribal conflicts beset farmers in Burundi, and widespread alcoholism and a long history of imposed change and control from outsiders have left few Hopi who continue the traditions of their elders. Everywhere, the pressures of new cash economies and competition for scarce resources create poverty where before there may have been enough. But beneath the hardships are examples of enduring qualities and techniques, threads that connect all true earth dwellers whether they are Peruvian potato farmers or Chinese rice growers.

First, they work with their land. They are always on it, walking it, touching it. There is a farmer's saying that "the best fertilizer is the farmer's footsteps on the field." I remember my Hopi friend describing the way he visits his fields at night, walking up and down the rows, singing to his corn.

In traditional agricultural communities, there is a careful balance of hands to acres, an appropriate scale that allows for intimacy with the land, the crops, and the animals. In the fields of modern American farms one person may be responsible for the management of thousands of acres, a fleeting glimpse from a pickup truck offering too little information to aid in careful stewardship and management.

Traditional farmers take all, but no more, than a generous earth can give. They use and tend every inch and often draw forth far greater yields on their land than modern farmers do on theirs. They understand the subtleties of rotation, of sensitive fertilization, and the appropriate use of hoe and plow.

They give back to the earth all they can—everything they have—in some cases, literally the shirts off their backs. I've seen Chinese peasants who will patch a piece of clothing till it can't hold another patch and then throw it into the compost. Human waste is recognized as a treasure, which it can be when properly treated. They nurture their scanty resources as a community, not just because community is pleasant in itself but for mutual survival. It's a very practical matter.

In traditional farming societies, food raising is a family affair. The knowledge is passed on, a sense of the wisdom of the earth. In Sicily I've seen four generations all working together harvesting or preparing field. And with the passing down of knowledge is also the passing down of seeds—seeds that contain a whole cultural history within their germ, representing local adaptation, disease and pest resistance, nutrition, and taste. The diversity of native food varieties has provided a key to the survival of those cultures, especially in areas where the climate and growing conditions are harsh.

And finally, traditional food growers take absolute responsibility for their own food—for virtually every mouthful they and their children eat. They don't leave that responsibility to supermarkets, chemical companies, the EPA, or the FDA.

Like the Peruvian potato that can survive and produce tubers at altitudes where we find it difficult to breathe or the Hopi corn that can push its way through ten inches of soil to bear fruit in the harsh desert landscape, traditional societies have also had to adapt to changes around them: economic, political, social, and environmental. That many of the practices of these cultures have survived under such pressure, some over millennia, is testimony to the power of shared traditional values, values that provide a cultural identity that allows them to persist.

If there is one thing the tenacity of these cultures has to offer us, it might be the example of a true and integrated ecological sensitivity, one that is manifested in the careful management of local resources and a fair exchange with the natural world around them. It is the ecological sensitivity, not intellectually derived but born out of the need to survive, that must become a part of our culture. Without it every attempt at environmental conservation or restoration will ultimately fail.

Life is a wheel
of elimination and decay,
nourishment and fertility.

—EDITOR

The first farmer was the first of many,
and all historic nobility rests
on possession and use of the land.

—EMERSON

One does not sell the earth
upon which the people walk.

—CRAZY HORSE

From to Soil to Plant to Plate

Bargyla Rateaver, Ph.D.

Why do we say that health begins in the soil?

Healthful nutrition is built on the fruits, vegetables and grains we eat—plants and their byproducts. But plants largely depend on the soil, so we recognize that nutrients originate in the soil. They originate directly, from humus and its minerals, and indirectly, from compounds produced by organisms that live in the soil.

The fundamental core of nutrition includes the major minerals, the complex carbohydrates, fats and proteins, together with special compounds needed in small amounts: vitamins, enzymes, coenzymes, essential fatty acids, energy/growth regulators, and trace elements. Production and application of all of these exist due to the soil, in which plants grow.

What is this vitally important soil?

The Complex Nature of Soil

Soil is not just dirt under our feet, but a whole world in itself, just as full of inhabitants as the world of humans, and as varied in life forms as the one in which we live. As Barry Commoner has said, "everything is connected to everything else," each world depending on the other in so many ways that it is impossible for us to comprehend the scope of its interconnections. We stand in awe at the variety, detail and complexity we see.

Real soil is the sum of three interdependent components: a base of minerals and organic compounds, the activities of microorganisms within this base, and an array of plant regulating compounds under the influence of water and air.

"Real soil consists of more than mineral particles, it is a furiously busy community of living things in stupendous variety. They range from viruses (huge molecules having some characterisitics of living organisms) to slime molds (creeping masses of naked protoplasm) to single-celled bacteria, algae and protozoa, to worms, rotifers, nematodes and multi-cellualr fungi, on up to earthworms, snails and slugs.

These organisms require moisture, respiratory fule and food. Water, organic material and the use of such supply these needs. Their excretions and secretions, their growth and physiological activity, their bodies and breakdown products of the organic matter, all add valuable traits to the soil, making it crumbly and well-drained, dark and velvety.

Real soil thus must have plenty of organic material together with the mineral elements and ideal conditions for soil life. It isn't real soil if you can't enjoy walking over it barefoot, however tender your feet are. It isn't real soil if you have to spade it up to make it loose. It isn't real soil if you can poke your fingers into it and tell whether the mineral particles are from sand or silt or clay.

Real soil is spongy and springy when you walk on it. Real soil will make a compact ball when you squeeze it in your hand, but crumbles apart at a touch. Real soil you can dig with your hands, and you can punch your closed fist right through it. When you brush off your hands, it leaves them clean. All you need of such stuff is one acre, to grow all you could want for yourself and your family."[1]

Food from plants grown in real soil, nutritionally balanced and biologically active, offers nutritional advantages over other foods such as its higher quality, improved flavor and extended storage characteristics. These plants have such a high Brix level that in prolonged storage they will dehydrate rather than rot. They have a hunger satisfying property that only real soil's characteristics provide, the actual basis of our health.

Our Dependence On Soil

Let's look at just six nutrients that depend on the soil:

1) The major item of our nutritional dependency on the soil is protein, the basis of life, that allows us to incorporate nitrogen, as nucleic acids, into the DNA/RNA of our genes. We must eat protein and ex-

pect to get it from plants, since they use nitrogen to make amino acids for linking into proteins and a variety of other needs, such as manufacturing enzymes and chlorophyll.

However, we receive major dietary protein only from legume plants—beans and peas, or the flesh of animals that eat these plants. Plants, in turn, derive their nitrogen content from the air.

We know that the air is four-fifths nitrogen, N_2 Nitrogen is a relatively inert element, essentially lifeless and without power, activity or motion. It isn't like oxygen which is less stable and therefore easily joined with other elements. Consequently, the best way nitrogen can become active is by being joined with an active element, such as oxygen, to start its activity. Partnered with oxygen, it can be joined to hydrogen by certain bacteria which invade the root of a plant and spend the rest of their lives inside of it, taking nitrogen gas from the air through the roots and changing it gradually into a form the plant can use: amino acids, to join as the proteins we need to eat. This routine is known as nitrogen fixation.

Hunger for nitrogen is felt by soil microbes, because only the nitrogen-containing RNA/DNA make it possible to reproduce the cells which manufacture proteins for new life. We are wholly dependent upon these bacteria for their role in supplying us with the protein we must eat in order to live, grow, heal and reproduce.

There are two main types of these nitrogen-fixing bacteria. Some free-living bacteria live on the *surface* of roots. These take advantage of the root's organic compounds for their own nourishment, and to fix nitrogen right there.

There are also bacteria, free living or symbiotic, on leaf surfaces. These are also able to fix nitrogen by living on leaf exudates, dead cells, detritus, trichomes, cuticle waxes, cellulase and pectins. This process is made possible by guttation, dew, rain, exudates and leachates, high in carbohydrates, but low in nitrogen.

Additionally, in some tropical plants, nitrogen-fixing bacteria reside in both roots and on stems.

2) Another example of our dependency on the soil is our requirement for a spectrum of minerals, which come from the soil through the action of soil organisms.

One group by which we gain mineral nutrients is the mycorrhizae, special types of fungi that interact with nitrogen fixation to greatly increase the absorption of minerals. They start their action in the root tip region of the soil which is differentiated by its exceptionally large microbe population.

A plant has billions of root hairs, their length equaling tens of thousands of miles. The root tip, with its thousands of delicate, single-celled root hairs, grows through a special region of this environment, the mucigel, a voluminous, gelatinous matrix in which it is embedded.

Into this highly enriched soil region are dumped millions of microbial derivatives, as well as exudates from the root, consisting of proteins, sugars, vitamins and mineral complexes, tannins, and alkaloids, no longer needed by the shoot.

Here, soil organisms work continuously to break down organic substances and build them up, reorganizing them into *new* compounds that contain minerals. These reactions are multitudinous, occurring millions of times per second in every minute mucigel fraction and producing myriads of re-structured molecules. Root hairs are offered, and prefer to absorb, these whole molecule nutrients that are constantly being created by the microlife of the mucigel community.

As the main, mineral-offering components of the rhizosphere, the mycorrhizal fungi (particularly in phosphorus-deficient soil), are generally so numerous that their environment may well be called the "mycorrhizosphere."[2] They help root hairs pick up nutrients, as their hyphal threads can forage much farther than the root itself.

Not only phosphorus is absorbed, but also trace minerals and certain micronutrients that the root welcomes from the microbial utopia. The whole nutrient system is monitored by these valuable fungi. In return, the root offers synthesized nutrients, such as sugars and proteins, to the hungry fungus in an epitome of symbiosis.

3) It is an absolute requirement that minerals must be chelated—wrapped in protein—to move through our living tissue. Again, we are dependent on soil organisms for such action, as it is they that do the chelating.

Although some minerals come from the air through openings in the green tissue surfaces, it is from the roots that most minerals are absorbed. Root hairs, growing in the surrounding gelatinous mucigel, prefer to pick up whole molecule nutrients, and these second-hand, as the microorganisms break down whatever substances they find and re-organize them into new compounds. This includes the protein they use to wrap minerals into chelated molecules, which are now suitable to feed the root hairs. This is how we depend on soil microorganisms for the chelated state of the minerals our metabolism requires.

4) Vitamins are catalysts, and we are also dependent upon soil organisms for these essential nutrients. Not only do these organisms utilize the vitamins given off to the air by plants, but they also produce them, and are thereby responsible for a direct effect on plant growth. Actinomycetes produce vitamin B_{12}, as few plants can. Certain algae secrete ascorbic acid.

5) We depend on soil organisms' catalytic activity by enzymes to insure the fertility that generally provides us with healthful food. The enzymes present in the soil generally correspond to its level of fertility. Many are found in the top soil horizons, where the majority of micro-organisms work (particularly the actinomycetes bacteria which directly excrete enzymes) and where fulvic acids stimulate enzyme formation. No cell reaction can occur unless the particular enzyme for that cell is present and ready to react, at optimum temperature and pH, so it can repeat this reaction hundreds of thousands of times each second. Ladd remarks that the contributions from enzymes of microbial origin are considered to be of great importance, and are enhanced under conditions favoring microbial growth and turnover."[3]

Once incorporated into plant tissues and assimilated into the body as food, enzymes can have a variety of roles in human digestion and metabolism. For example, the common enzyme phosphatase assists in the absorption of phosphorus and calcium from our food.

6) Our most comprehensive dependency is based on humus, the overall end product of soil metabolism that provides humic and fulvic acids.[4] These acids are involved in almost everything that goes on in organic soil. In solution, they directly or indirectly affect plant metabolism—positive effects of humus acids on DNA in the plant cell nucleus and RNA in the plant cell cytoplasm. These effects are directed by genes, since humic and fulvic acids contain components that affect membrane functions.

In mineral complexing and chelating, it is the water-soluble fulvic acids that efficiently make the new structures.

The plants we depend on for food require growth regulators controlling their development: gibberellins, auxins and cytokinins, and here too humic and fulvic acids play a role, encouraging production of many core molecules in numerous ways.

Kononova mentions that small fulvic acids move to the shoots of plants through the water-conducting tissue (xylem) and activate enzyme systems there, influencing respiration: when oxygen becomes insufficient, addition of these acids enables the plant to overcome the oxygen shortage.[5]

Conclusion

Human nutrition depends on all these nutrients that come from living soil. Even meat and dairy products come from animals which eat plants grown in the soil; therefore all foods ultimately come from the soil.

Plants need the same nitrogen, minerals and organic compounds that we need and depend on the richness of the soil community organisms for these nutrients. It is clear that we, then, who depend on plants for our nourishment, are ultimately dependent on the soil where the life routines begin.

This is the basis of health and nutrition through the living soil created by organic agriculture.

Everything is not food for man,
and what may be food for him
is not equally suitable.

—ROUSSEAU

Earth's increase, foison plenty,
Barns and garners never empty,
Vines with clustering bunches growing,
Plants with goodly burden bowing;

Spring comes to you at the farthest
In the very end of harvest!
Scarcity and want shall shun you;
Ceres blessing so is on you.

—SHAKESPEARE

One of the basic principles of organic gardening
is to feed the soil and let the soil feed the plants;
then the plants can feed you.

—SHEPHERD OGDEN

Biodynamic Farming*
and Society

HERBERT H. KOEPF, PH.D.

EXCERPTS FROM *THE BIODYNAMIC FARM*, ANTHROPOSOPHIC PRESS, HUDSON, NY 1989. USED BY PERMISSION OF ANTHROPOSOPHIC PRESS.

During the last forty years or so, conventional farming has followed a course that is radically different from what biodynamic and many organic farmers do. Science has provided the technology; economic forces have provided the drive. Specialized farms in specialized production zones, bigger farms, larger implements to reduce the need for human labor, and large amounts of external inputs are some of the tools by which farmers have tried to increase their income, and to mitigate the rising cost of labor and industrial goods. Government incentives have supported this development. Large-scale corporate production is the logical next step on this road. The social costs of these systems have now become a concern of a wider public. Finally, the 1980s have revealed an economic impasse for the farmer and his family.

In spite of this general economic and social climate, the number of farms changing to biodynamic methods increase steadily. By now biodynamics is applied in a number of very different natural, economic, and social settings. The farmers, gardeners, advisers, and re-

---

*Editor's note: The Biodynamic approach to agriculture is based upon the teachings of the German philosopher-scientist, Dr. Rudolph Steiner (1861-1925). This aspect of his philosophy continues to be practiced around the world as a practical model for sustainable agriculture

searchers involved in biodynamic work did not have the gigantic infrastructure of research, extension services, training, and government help that made conventional farming what it is. Nevertheless, biodynamic farmers are progressive. Most of them have completed some kind of formal training, and they do not disregard the up-to-date biological and technical information taught in colleges or assembled in university libraries. However, they use this information selectively toward biodynamic goals. By using suitable farm machinery, improved methods of cultivation, improved building designs, proper cultivation, and so on, they keep pace with the general development. Needless to say, they have to pay attention to economic realities, but their ultimate goal is a larger one. Let us now touch on some of the human issues, such as motivation, goals, social attitudes, and education that are so important for biodynamics and for leading agriculture into the future.

Motivation

What feeds the motives of biodynamic farmers? This question was touched on in the introductory remarks to this book. Their concern is to take proper care of the soil and all the creatures under their responsibility.

In part this feeling is a cultural heritage. The social forms and human values of traditional agriculture strengthened the feeling of responsibility for the land and what grows on it. But powerful forces are active that erode such attitudes. Nowadays many of those who grow up in a rural district expect the city to offer them a more rewarding life. On the other hand, there is a smaller but slowly growing number of young people who try to live a meaningful life on the land. They come from urban backgrounds. Their search is not always carried by a realistic image of farming or gardening, but it is genuine and sincere. The strong ones meet the challenge, but many others have to leave. One encounters in our time many individual human destinies that have to find their way to the hardships and rewards of a rural life. An understanding of these individuals reveals that ultimately the decision to choose this work comes from within. Economic circumstances may assist the decision, but more often they are serious constraints and may prevent a person from doing what he or she really wants to do. The resolve to be a farmer and to stay with it must be rooted in layers of the human being of which economics is merely a part.

A materialistic world view can never kindle the motivation for a way of farming in harmony with life proper. Yet such harmony is a prerequisite if destructive exploitation is to be avoided. It can grow out of a spiritual understanding of living nature. To warn people that they must not destroy the very basis that sustains the life of all is not enough. A spiritual outlook is needed. Modern science investigates soils and plants and discovers innumerable material details that are worth knowing. These also put man in a position to manipulate many processes from outside, as it were. But at the same time, they make people blind to the essential life in the kingdoms of nature.

Human beings share with minerals a physical body, with plants a living body, and with animals an ensouled existence. Human beings rise above all these kingdoms because they are capable of observing and consciously grasping in thought the manifestations of the forces of life. They observe how the seed germinates and how the shoot unfolds in air and light. In the warmth of the sun the process hastens to complete the cycle in flowering and seed formation. Before the eye and mind of the human being, the invisible plant enters into visibility and withdraws again, leaving behind the minute germ embedded in the seed. This transformation of forms and substances is consistent, every step leads to the next. But that totality never stands before our eyes as a single physical appearance. It is only the power of thought that can actively mold into a telling picture what would otherwise remain fragmented appearances occurring in time. In the human being the life process becomes conscious and coherent. One participates in its progress. It does not escape the mind that to view this process as something standing by itself would not be true. This would be an abstraction alienated from reality, because in reality each plant is a part of the immense life that spreads through the soil, that moves in the air, and pulsates through day and night, summer and winter. The earthly and cosmic surroundings are what bring the potential life in the seed to its specific manifestation.

Human beings similarly seek to understand animals and their behaviors in a deeper way. From the way in which they move and act, it is obvious that animals share with us a conscious life of pain and pleasure, desire and satisfaction. How they are formed and react reveals wisdom. In a strange way they are also fixed and limited in their daily routine and respond to influences from outside, although they are bound in their behavioral pattern. Daily work keeps the farmer in close touch with living and ensouled nature, with her individual creatures, and with the community at large. To meet this essential reality helps farmers fashion their work. This reality is the basis for ethical values. It is a dimension of a farmer's life that must not get drowned by actual or alleged economic necessities.

Stewardship

The major part of a nation's soil is used to produce food, feed, and fiber. Agricultural systems that use up soil fertility for transient gains deprive the country and future generations of their most important resource. Modern conventional farming shows many characteristics of such systems. Apart from growing food and earning a living for their families, farmers should be in a position to act as stewards of the national soil. For most farmers, this is a genuine desire. Historically, however, soil destruction has usually prevailed. One need only look at the countries on the Mediterranean Sea now; formerly they produced all the wheat Rome needed. Until recently one could argue that somewhere in this country or elsewhere on the earth new land could still be found and reclaimed. This time is past. Destroying land for short-term gains must now come to an end, even in those areas where some additional land might be found for farming or for speculative gain.

There is yet another factor affecting the work of the farmer. A generation or two ago, the average good farmer may not have been a wealthy man. However, he was in a rather secure position. He earned enough money to gradually pay for the farm he had bought with relatively little cash at hand and occasionally to buy some additional land. This has changed. The long-term stability of farming is at risk. Land has become too expensive to pay for it by farming. The monetary situation of the majority of all farms calls for continued adjustments to the market, regardless of the negative effects on lasting fertility. Current economic pressures do not allow farmers to do as much for conservation as they would wish. On the other hand, many farmers chose maximum profit as the goal of their farming enterprises and thus neglected conservation measures when they could have afforded them.

Rural and Urban Interface

A third structural change in our food system has taken place in recent times. There is no longer a close link between the primary producer of the food and his urban consumers. A huge system of transportation, processing, and distribution has established itself between consumers and producers. The relationship has changed from a very personal to an anonymous one. Many people are hardly aware that there should be a relationship at all. Roadside markets offering home-grown and home-processed goods are an exception. By and large the outer and inner distance between the land and the urban consumer has become very great.

As stewards of the land, farmers fulfill a function for the common weal. Economic pressures can prevent them from properly meeting this task, and the urban population may hardly know about it. This is a brief description of a rather complex situation. Granted, the food system in industrialized countries provides more foodstuffs in a greater variety all year round for more people than ever before, but one must not turn a blind eye to its negative aspects.

New Roads

Every farmer who practices sustainable husbandry makes an individual contribution to a healthier system. But more needs to be done. In the biodynamic movement a number of individual initiatives are in progress that address the questions of land ownership, working in groups, and furthering relevant relationships between the agricultural sector and other groups in our society.

The private ownership of land is a relatively recent occurrence in human history. In former times, the land was viewed as God-given and was held as a common resource for the people. Authorities such as the tribe, the landlord, the crown, and the church administered the use of the land. With the dawn of our modern age, humanity strove for independence and freedom for all members of society. This mode of consciousness has its corollary in the private ownership of land and, for that matter, of other means of production as well. Land can be used by human beings, and we have the possibility of maintaining or destroying it in the pursuit of our economic goals. The power of the authorities of older times who used to regulate land use has now been taken over by money, by individual rights, and by governmental objectives. The modern ecological crisis is partly the result of this change. There has rarely ever been harmony between the requirements of sustainable agriculture and the demands made by society. Yet in our time, more than ever before in history, it has become obvious that the people who actually take the necessary steps to preserve or improve long-term fertility should be those who cultivate the land. In place of the authorities of the past, the free decision of individuals or groups must now put this basic principle into practice. In the larger context of the situation, the success of such farmers will ultimately depend on the relationship other sections of society find to the land.

In view of the hard realities of economic life this sounds like wishful thinking. Nevertheless, a number of initiatives are in progress, arising from biodynamic work or related to it, that are putting into practice the idea that tillable soil should not be a commodity. The land they hold is no longer treated as a private asset. It cannot be sold, inherited, or even used as a security. Projects registered as an "Agricultural Community" or "Agricultural Research Society," etc., share such principles and objectives. Such projects are organized according to the economic and human situation particular to each case. The farm as an individuality, in the social as well as the ecological sense, is the underlying image. The emphasis is on bringing farmers and nonfarmers who share spiritual and social goals into a working relationship. These people are jointly responsible for the capital and the means of production that are then put at the disposal of those who work on the farm.

The land put into the organization (which is usually a nonprofit land trust) is either purchased or donated. Farmers who take the step to make their land available usually live on the farm and enjoy its fruits for their lifetime. But the status of the land will never change, not even when they pass away.

The individuals who actually do the farming are free to shape their activity as they think best. Together with the landholding organization, they are coresponsible for the agricultural, economic, and social development of the business. Both parties develop the long-term policy for work, finances, and agricultural and cultural activities. The partners enter into arrangements tailored to specific conditions and their potential.

It is obvious that these projects by their very nature are likely to attract additional activities, such as processing, milling, baking, cheese making, canning, etc.; marketing usually stimulates diversification in the production program, e.g., vegetable production. But other activities such as educational and curative work have also been taken up in a number of cases. Working in groups is the obvious foundation for this kind of setup. In some, but not in all respects, these projects are similar to those in which curative or educational homes also own land.

All human beings need food, clothing, and other material things to sustain their physical existence. Thus, in an ideal-realistic sense everybody "owns," but is also "individually responsible" for, a proportional share of the land and, in fact, of the means of production. To put this idea into practice "Agricultural Communities" are formed and incorporated that issue shares in the land and the agricultural operation. This capital is used to develop the farm and its affiliated enterprises and to supply the general market with goods. Those who are immediately responsible for the farming and the business are answerable to the whole group. Each in turn shares the financial implications for the sound development of the project and for the material and cultural life of those who work it.

This concise description should make clear that those projects are very much built on the initiatives, the creative work, and the responsible will of the individuals who join in. By now, more than a dozen of these projects have been in progress for fifteen years or longer. Their number is considerably larger if homes for curative education and similar institutions are included.

Training in Biodynamic Farming and Gardening must go beyond learning an efficient technology. Its goals include a deeper understanding of the workings of living nature and human development. In the introductory chapter the significance of experience, skills, and know-how was emphasized. These are not just prerequisites for practicing successful farming. They are necessary for the farmer who wants to mold his ideals and the physical necessities of farming into a unity. Farming's unique quality is to offer individuals a way to unite ideals and practice. The vocations of teachers, doctors, and a few other professions lend themselves to such development as well, but most people have to divide their time between their jobs and their avocational cultural endeavors and hobbies.

In the biodynamic movement various training programs are operative. These programs all stress the importance of practical experience acquired by working full-time through the cycle of the year. This experience should be gathered by working for several years on more than one farm. It goes without saying that the biodynamic schools listed in Appendix 2 give due attention to teaching plant and animal husbandry in a technical sense though in the context of the biodynamic method; yet spiritual and cultural values are also very prominent in their programs. A study of humanity and the kingdoms of nature in the light of the science of the spirit, of the forces working in the earthly realm and in the cosmic expanses, are components of the curriculum. Later on this will give the students strength and advisory jobs, and also for building relevant contacts with their fellow farmers.

During his lectures on agriculture Rudolf Steiner found the time early in the morning to address a group of younger men and women. Some of them were future farmers. He spoke about the search of the younger generation, their wanting to reach beyond the sterile materialistic world view of modern times. "You are seeking the spirit in nature," he said. This search is central to what biodynamic farmers and gardeners strive to accomplish. Its general application creates a form of agriculture that truly serves the earth and humanity.

When Rudolf Steiner gave the agriculture lectures described above, he also wrote a report on what he was doing. According to Steiner, his lectures were addressing: "practical points that add to what one has gained by practical experience and scientific research, what from a spiritual aspect can be said about (agricultural) matters."

Steiner's approach can be called *qualitative-ecological* in contrast to the *analytical-quantitative* approach of conventional science. "Ecological" is here meant to embrace all the earthly and cosmic forces that form life. Biodynamics puts qualitative ecological principles into practice in the following ways:

Biodynamic farms are formed in the image of an organism. They have a site-adapted and balanced combination of plant and animal husbandry. Biodynamic farms attempt to be self-sufficient with respect to manures and feed-stuffs. Within the totality of the farm, human capabilities and needs and marketing potential get due attention.

Production is sustainable because it is based on cropping and manuring systems that preserve and improve the productivity of the soil. Farm-produced manures are carefully collected and handled to recycle nutrients. If necessary, slowly soluble minerals are used.

Disease and pest control are primarily based on the preventative potential of the system, i.e., a combination of enterprises, and also on inoffensive substances. Weed control is achieved by rotating crops and by cultivation. Specific dynamic measures to regulate weeds and pests are being developed and are to some extent already in use.

Feed for livestock is mostly produced on the farm, and the production of seedstocks is adapted to the system and the site.

The life processes in the soil, plants and manure are regulated and stimulated by dynamic measures. This is achieved by using small quantities of preparations made from herbs and other substances.

Consideration is given to subtle processes and interactions. These interactions include those of plant and animal communities, insect and bird life, moist biotopes, wooded and agricultural land, hedges, and other ecological niches. The general life of nature and plant life in particular are considered to be immersed in a wider environment including the cosmic realm surrounding the earth. The solar year rhythm and other bio-chrono-logical rhythms are considered important for the growth and quality of produce.

Stable and satisfactory economic returns can be provided by bio-dynamic systems. From the stand point of national economy, the biodynamic farm produces optimum results while wisely managing resources and energy. The biodynamic farm does not pollute because it avoids using a host of questionable agricultural chemicals.

The macro-ecological effects of the layout and management of biodynamic farms are the maximum possible conservation of soils, the quality of water bodies, the enhanced health of wildlife, and the improved quality of the rural environment.

Human values and a unity between a world view and motivation are furthered by a caring approach based on giving and taking.

A longing in the hearts and minds of many people living in our technically and economically oriented society has made itself heard since the 1960s. Many are looking for a way of life the unites and heals rather than for one that tends to isolate people or split them into interest groups. Many of these people are also interested in alternative agriculture. However, such longings may create their own constraints unless a modern, scientifically sound, spiritual knowledge of man and nature forms a firm basis for a sensitive and ethical approach. Biodynamics is based on such an approach.

One animal is devoted exclusively
to the humus production
—the earthworm.

—Dr. Ehrenfried Pfeiffer

So long as one feeds on food from unhealthy soil,
the spirit will lack the stamina to free itself
from the prison of the body.

—Rudolf Steiner

Man shapes himself through decisions
that shape his environment.

—Rene Du Bois

Towards a Sustainable Agriculture—The Living Soil

Lady Eve Balfour

The following address was given by Lady Balfour to an IFOAM conference in Switzerland in 1977. Reproduced with permission from the Organic Gardening and Farming Society of Tasmania Inc.

In order to set the scene for this historic conference, and for the benefit of the younger participants, I think it might be helpful to start by sketching, briefly, the origins and development of the, now worldwide, organic movement. After that I propose to explain how my own involvement in the movement led to the so-called 'Haughley Experiment', and outline the contribution which that experiment made towards today's recognition of the importance of ecological awareness in Agriculture. Finally I want to share with you some of my thoughts on what I believe should be our approach, both philosophical and pragmatic, in working for a Sustainable Agriculture.

I do not know where or when the ideas that have brought us together here were first called a movement, but I have little doubt that the main inspiration derived from the work of the early research pioneers in the first quarter of this century, though this is not to discount the influence of one of the most important, who was even earlier, namely Rudolf Steiner.

Those I particularly have in mind were: in the medical field, Sir Robert McCarrison, Drs. Francis Pottinger Jnr. and Weston Price, and in the agricultural field, Sir Albert Howard, Dr. William Albrecht, and Dr. E. Pfeiffer.

Following these, and overlapping with them to a certain extent, came another wave of giants—men like Dr. George Scott-Williamson, Dr. Lionel Picton, Dr. Dendy, Prof. Barry Commoner and the courageous Rachel Carson, and among the list of departed great ones, I must, sadly, now add Dr. Schumacher.

These pioneers had one thing in common- they were what we should now call Ecologists. They all succeeded in breaking away from the narrow confines of the preconceived ideas that dominated the scientific thinking of their day. They looked at the living world from a new perspective- they also asked new questions. Instead of the contemporary obsession with disease and its causes, they set out to discover the causes of Health. This led inevitably to an awareness of wholeness (the two words after all, have the same origin) and to a gradual understanding that all life is one.

Although I started farming in Suffolk in 1919 my own interest in the ecological approach only began in the early 1920's. By that time local societies had been formed in more than one country to promote organic husbandry and whole food, though I was not aware of this until 1945 when plans were under way for forming the Soil Association, the first society in the movement aiming at a world membership, and with research high on its list of priorities, which brings me to the Haughley Experiment.

This was started in 1939 on my farm and taken over by the Soil Association in 1947 which for the next 25 years directed and sponsored it. This pioneering experiment was the first ecologically designed agricultural research project, on a full farm scale. It was set up to fill a gap in the evidence on which the claims for the benefits of organic husbandry were based. It was decided that the only way to achieve this was to observe and study nutrition cycles, functioning as a whole, under contrasting methods of land use, but on the same soil and under the same management, the purpose being to assess what effect, if any, the different soil treatments had on the biological quality of the produce grown thereon, including its nutritive value as revealed through its animal consumers. This had never been done before.

Three side-by-side units of land were established, each large enough to operate a full farm rotation, so that the food-chains involved—soil—plant—animal and back to the soil, could be studied as they functioned through successive rotational cycles, involving many generations of plants and animals, in order that interdependencies between soil, plant and animal, and also any cumulative effects could manifest.

In order that you may understand the significance of some of the results I cannot avoid a short summary of how these units were operated. One was a stockless arable farm which for the purpose of this talk I shall ignore—the other two were both ley farms (temporary pasture alternating with arable) operating the same rotation. Each carried a herd of dairy cows, a flock of poultry and a small flock of sheep. All livestock was fed exclusively on the produce of its own unit, replacements were home bred and cereal and pulse crops raised from home-grown seed. All wastes of crops and stock were returned only to its own unit. Only livestock products and surplus animals were sold off the farm. All crops were put through the animals. On one of these two comparable units supplementary chemical fertilizers were used, as well as herbicides, insecticides and fungicides when thought necessary. This unit was called the Mixed Section.

On the other unit, called the Organic Section, no chemicals were used. It was thus entirely dependent on its own biological fertility. As nearly as possible a closed cycle was maintained so that a minimum of unknown factors should be introduced into the food chain to confuse the issue.

You can see, I expect, why such an exploration into the unknown was left to the private enterprise of a charitable society with small resources. It was at total variance with the fragmentary techniques of orthodox agricultural research, which is based on randomized small plots—a technique quite incapable of throwing any light on biological interdependencies in a functioning whole. The establishment of the day even went so far as to declare that there was no case to investigate—they were particularly critical of the closed system on the organic section, yet most of the significant findings were the outcome of this, and would not have been revealed without it. I will attempt to summarize a few of the more important findings, concentrating on those that have special relevance for the subject matter of this conference.

In addition to carefully recorded field observations, an extensive range of sample analyses (soil and products) was carried out by the consultant bio-chemist, Dr. R.F. Milton. These included analyses for available plant nutrients in every field every month for a period of over 10 years.

The outcome of this huge number of individual analyses, running into thousands, was a new discovery. It was one of the most important single findings to come out of the experiment, because it was so conclusive and, surprisingly, hitherto unsuspected by orthodox agricultural chemists—namely that the levels of available minerals in the soil fluctuate according to the season, maximum levels coinciding with the time of maximum plant demand. These fluctuations were far more marked on the Organic Section than on the other two, where, moreover, they could be partly related to fertilizer application.

On the Organic Section, which received no fertilizers, the fluctuation was so marked that, for example, in the field with the highest humus content and the longest history of no chemicals, as much as 10 times more available phosphate has been recorded in the growing period of the year than in the dormant period. Potash and nitrogen followed the same general pattern. It was clear, from the fact of the closed cycle, that this seasonal release of minerals could only have been brought about by biological agencies, and it appears to be a natural action-pattern of a biologically active soil.

When this finding was first published it was taken up by a Scottish University, repeated, confirmed, and is now generally accepted. Previously it had been assumed that a single spot analysis at any time of year could show what the soil required.

The many different chemical analyses, carried out on crops and livestock products, revealed no consistent or significant differences between the sections, other than the usually higher water content of the chemically grown fodder. Seasonal variations, and those between fields in the same section, often exceeded average sectional differences. But this lack of difference was in itself significant in that on the organic section, receiving no added minerals, the analysis of soil and crops showed a nutrient status that remained consistently as high as that of the others.

This indicates how little of the minerals applied as fertilizers are recovered in crops, and is important in relation to the purpose of this conference. Dr. Milton has summed it up thus: 'The analytical work carried out in connection with the Haughley Experiment has shown how wasteful of natural resources is modern commercial farming and how with a closed-cycle technique nutrients are recycled and moreover become available in situ provided that an ecological approach is made to the methods of cultivation and farm management.

Although analytical differences between the sections was negligible, there were functional differences of some significance, such as the relative freedom from insect pest damage of the organic section crops, and the longer working life of its livestock. A number of the functional differences noted threw up unanswered questions and so point the directions for useful future research.

Three examples must serve to illustrate what I mean:

1. In spite of the mixed section receiving no less organic return than its organic counterpart it could be clearly demonstrated that its fields had become dependent on their fertilizer supplements in a manner suggestive of drug addiction. By contrast the organic fields developed an increasing biological vigor which enabled them to be self-supporting. Had we not operated the closed cycle policy, this surprising result would almost certainly have been attributed to whatever importation had taken place. I shall be referring later to research work carried out during the last year and not yet published in detail that may provide at least a partial explanation for this and my next example.

2. A consistent finding, particularly with autumn sown cereals, was a visual observation of an apparently much delayed growth in the early stages on the Organic Section. Further examination, however, showed that in this initial period the plant in an organic environment is 'concentrating' (if I may so put it) on establishing a vigorous root system. Having done so, but not before, it is ready to make top growth (i.e. the behavior pattern of growth is quite different to that of plants growing in a chemical or 'mixed' environment). This interpretation is supported by the fact that before the end of the growing season the 'organic' crops caught up the others and, as I have stated, remained able to look after themselves.

3. With the livestock, the temperament of the animals composing the herds and flocks exhibited sectional differences, those belonging to the organic section being noticeably more contented. Our findings also confirmed the many reports received from organic farmers in different parts of the world, that a given output of animal products—

milk, meat, eggs etc. required from 12-15% less input of food when this was grown organically.

At Haughley, for example, though the organic herbal leys were of clearly sparser growth than the much lusher mixed-section leys, the cows on the former gave, over a 20 year period, around 15% more milk than the other. (To forestall the obvious comment, we were able to show that this contrast was not due to a genetic factor.)

Once more this finding is relevant to any discussion about an alternative and sustainable agriculture, and this is what I now want to talk about. To start with, I want to answer three widely held objections to the idea that organic farming on a world scale can ever be possible.

The most frequently heard argument is that intensive chemical farming provides the only hope of feeding the expanding world population and has therefore to be accepted whether we like it or not. To me it seems probable that the exact opposite could prove to be the case, and that it is an alternative and largely organic agriculture that will be forced upon us whether we like it or not. This is because, as is becoming increasingly apparent, the days of the former are numbered. One reason is the enormous demands on the world's non-renewable resources of energy made by our Western life-style in general and modern farming techniques in particular. Another is that modern methods are putting strains on the biota which is causing it to collapse.

Thus it is only common sense to look at alternatives and in all seriousness study their potential viability.

It is not yet, however, generally accepted that the days of our present methods and behavior are numbered. Even where it is, it is too often regarded as a long term problem which must not be allowed to obscure the immediate problem, namely the need to increase quantitative food production now. Here it is argued that organic farming is less efficient, that it has to rely on re-cycling which is wasteful, so that were it to be adopted, world food production would inevitably be lower, particularly production of protein, at a time when what we need is to produce ever more per acre.

To this I would like to point out three things:

1. A common view among nutritionists today is that the amount of protein (especially animal protein) hitherto thought to be required by

man has been greatly over- estimated. (Organic farmers have found this also to be true for livestock).

2. There need be little loss in re-cycling if we did not waste so much.

3. Certainly we need to produce more per acre. Unfortunately the yardstick of modern economics is to measure the efficiency by production per man.

Labor-intensive small units will always be able to produce spectacularly more per acre than the large mechanized farms, apart from the finding that organically grown food goes further. When the inevitable change in life-style takes place I predict that we shall find it easier to feed the world population than we think, perhaps easier than now because Western Nations will presumably have become less gluttonous. I predict also that we shall all be healthier!

We still hear, though less frequently than we used to, the argument that there is no scientific basis for advocating exclusive use of organic manures, such as FYM and compost, because 'there is absolutely no difference between a plant nutrient contained in organic materials and the same nutrient in in-organic chemical form.' There may be no chemical, or other easily analyzable difference, but there is a demonstrable functional difference. Anything having an effect on root distribution, for example, may have an effect on plant nutrition because it will influence the volume of soil explored.

Thus good soil structure in depth, such as is obtained in a biologically active soil, can improve productivity simply by increasing the depth of soil exploited for water and nutrients. There is now well documented scientific evidence that fertilizer concentrations of N and P have an influence on localized root branching. They induce it at the expense of deep rooting exploration. This could well lead to luxury uptakes of N and P linked to inadequate uptake of other nutrients.

There are implications in this for nutrient unbalance in the crop and thereby some risk of nutrient unbalance in the animals and humans feeding upon it. If root activity is a factor in the development and maintenance of soil structure, there are also implications in this for the overall pattern of soil development.

This is the work I was referring to earlier as possibly throwing light on some Haughley findings. (A reference to it is M.C. Drew Ag. Research Council Letcome Laboratory Annual Report for 1975.63-1976).

In a biologically active soil, which implies one adequately provided with organic matter and natural rock minerals, the latter are released as the plants want them. Moreover, the roots are presented with a complete diet from which they can pick and choose.

Plants are highly selective in such circumstances, hence the value of some of the deep rooting weeds (which the organic farmer calls herbs when he sows them deliberately). Normal chemical fertilizers, apart from the disadvantage just mentioned are far too simple: A plant's mineral requirements are many times wider in range. By giving only two or three which stimulate bulk growth, others, equally important, are exhausted or locked up in the immediate neighborhood of the rhizosphere thus leading, as already mentioned, to unbalanced nutrition of the plant and, often through their solubility, to serious environmental pollution.

Plant nutrients do not, as was once taught, all have to be reduced to simple inorganic solutions in order to be absorbed. Plants can ingest quite complex organic molecules, unbroken. The history of D.D.T. provides irrefutable evidence for this. So do such symbiotic mechanisms as mycorrhizal association, whereby the plant may well derive some nutrient equivalent to vitamins in animal nutrition.

A possible additional factor for which, I readily admit, there is at present no scientific proof but which seems to me to provide an interpretation consistent with many observations, is that in nature's foodchains, a plant's normal method of mineral intake is not direct but second-hand, the mineral plant-foods being, as it were, by- products of the activity of the soil micro-flora and other members of the soil population.

Such by-products have a far more complex and comprehensive formula than N, P and K and moreover are living substances. Inorganic chemicals are inert. A food-chain is not only a material circuit, but also an energy circuit. Soil fertility has been defined as the capacity of soil to receive, store and transmit energy. A substance may be the same chemically but very different as a conductor of living energy. The hypothesis is that the energy manifesting in birth, growth, reproduction, death, decay and rebirth, can only flow through channels composed of living cells, and that when the flow is interrupted by inert matter it can be short-circuited with consequent damage to some part of the food-chain, not necessarily where the block occurred. The Anthroposophical Society's Research establishment at Dornach in this country (Switzerland) has provided some evidence in support of such a view.

I would like to see much more research undertaken in this field.

Now I want to put forward what I believe our aims should be in evolving a sustainable agriculture, and then, finally, pass on to you some thoughts on organic farming as I see it.

The criteria for a sustainable agriculture can be summed up in one word—permanence, which means adopting techniques that maintain soil fertility indefinitely; that utilize, as far as possible, only renewable resources; that do not grossly pollute the environment; and that foster life energy (or if preferred biological activity) within the soil and throughout the cycles of all the involved food-chains.

This is what biological husbandry sets out to attempt—with an increasing degree of understanding and success among its practitioners. Throughout the world, as a result of their own experience, these sincerely believe that they can offer a genuine and viable alternative agriculture, capable of solving many of the problems of mankind. This possibility, as well as the need for it, is becoming increasingly recognized in academic and scientific circles.

I am often asked how, in a broad sense, I define Organic Farming as opposed to conventional farming. Though I prefer the term biological husbandry because of its emphasis on life, the short answer is balance; however I think it is necessary to amplify a little.

Contrary to the views held by some, I am sure that the techniques of organic farming cannot be imprisoned in a rigid set of rules. They depend essentially on the outlook of the farmer. Without a positive and ecological approach it is not possible to farm organically. The approach of the modern conventional farmer is negative, narrow and fragmentary, and consequently produces imbalance. His attitude to 'pests' and 'weeds', for example, is to regard them as enemies to be killed—if possible exterminated. When he attacks them with lethal chemicals he seldom gives a thought to the effect this may have on the food supply or habitat of other forms of wildlife among whom he has many more friends than foes. The predatory insects and the insectivorous birds are obvious examples.

The attitude of the organic farmer, who has trained himself to think ecologically, is different. He tries to see the living world as a whole. He regards so-called pests and weeds as part of the natural pattern of the Biota, probably necessary to its stability and permanence, to be utilized rather than attacked. Throughout his operations he endeavors to achieve his objective by co-operating with natural agencies in place of relying on man-made substitutes. He studies what appear to be nature's rules—as manifested in a healthy wilderness—and attempts to adapt them to his own farm needs, instead of flouting them.

One of the first things he will notice about a natural eco-system such as a Wilderness or a Natural Forest is Balance and Stability. The innumerable different species of fauna and flora that go to make up such a community achieve, as a result of their interdependence, whether in co-operation or competition, collective immortality. Seldom, if ever, is any species eliminated; seldom, if ever, does any species multiply to pest proportions. Thus the organic farmer, if he has a crop badly attacked by some pest, let us say, (and this can happen, even to organic farmers!) recognizes that this is a symptom of imbalance in his local environment, and he first looks to see if some faulty technique of his own has been responsible—often it has.

This does not mean that he can always avoid emergency remedial measures but these he employs only when there is a real emergency, not as a routine. He strives instead to bring about biological balance, and it is remarkable the extent to which organic farmers and growers do in fact achieve this. I could give you several examples, but one must suffice.

Some years ago a large scale organic commercial grower of my acquaintance, growing vegetables, fruit and flowers was visited by a team of scientists from Cambridge University—they included plant pathologists and entomologists. They knew it was an unsprayed holding and they came looking for disease and pests. They found isolated examples of everything they expected to find, but, as they put it, they failed to find a single case of crop damage.

Besides biological balance, the ecologically minded organic farmer takes note of, and tries to apply, other apparent biological roles. For example, nature's diversity of species he adapts through rotations, under-sowing, and avoiding monoculture of crops or animals. Nature's habit of filtering sunlight and rain through some form of protective soil cover he adapts by such practices as cover-cropping and mulching. Top soil on the top appears to be nature's plan. Organic matter is always deposited on the surface. It is left to the earthworms and some insects to take it below. The organic farmer also puts his compost and farmyard manure on, or very near, the surface and in carrying out mechanical cultivations keeps soil-inversion to a minimum, the tine cultivator being preferred to the plough.

Nature's highly efficient re-cycling system ensures provision of living food for all organisms in the food chain from soil bacteria and fungi to large fauna; the organic farmer therefore lays great stress on the conservation and return to the soil of all organic residues. His aim is to feed and to assist proliferation of the soil population and to leave it to feed the crop.

Finally, and of equal importance, he notes, and tries to reproduce, the almost perfect structure of a biologically active soil which alone ensures the three most important characteristics of a fertile soil—good aeration, water-holding capacity, and free drainage.

It is quite astonishing the extent to which this all-important property of good soil is neglected in modern agriculture. Poor soil structure leads to imbalance between water and air in the pore spaces of the soil. Many apparent mineral or trace mineral deficiencies in the soil turn out to be oxygen deficiencies. When that is corrected the others disappear.

In most agricultural soils there is really plenty of mineral plant food for the nutritional requirements of plants, even when continuously cropped, if their roots are allowed to exploit it downwards. The key to this is good soil structure which is greatly influenced by the activity of earthworms. The techniques of modern farming tend to destroy good structure in a number of ways, such as by the impaction of heavy implements, by carrying out cultivations in unsuitable weather conditions, and by failure to provide sufficient organic food and/or a suitable lime status for the earthworm population.

All these faults are the outcome of failure to think ecologically—they are symptoms of a degree of fragmentation in our approach to the living world which has become a real threat to our survival. Throughout biological evolution, starting from single celled organisms right up to the complexity of rain forests, the process has been characterized by increasing diversity among species, lengthening of the food chains, and progressive enrichment of the environment.

For the first time in the history of the planet the actions of modern man appear to be putting this process into reverse. Whole species of fauna and flora are being eliminated, the food-chains are becoming shorter, and the environment progressively impoverished. It only takes a little imagination to picture what could happen if the trend continues.

What are we going to do about it? This is the real challenge for the International Federation of Organic Agriculture Movements, and in my view it is one of education. The Soil Association is doing an excellent pioneering job in adult education into the principles and practice of biological husbandry. It is now urgently necessary that a still wider aspect of ecology should also form part of the regular curriculum of all schools, starting at the primary stage. The trouble is we have first to teach the teachers, and here, I think, we must be agreed upon what we want to teach.

There are two motivations behind an ecological approach—one is based on self interest, however enlightened, i.e. when consideration for other species is taught solely because on that depends the survival of our own.

The other motivation springs from a sense that the biota is a whole, of which we are a part, and that the other species which compose it and helped to create it; are entitled to existence in their own right. This is the wholeness approach and it is my hope and belief that this is what we, as a federation, stand for.

If I am right, this means that we cannot escape from the ethical and spiritual values of life for they are part of wholeness. To ignore them and their implications would be to pursue another form of fragmentation. Therefore, I hold that what we have to teach is the attitude defined by Aldo Leopold as 'A Land Ethic.' This requires that we extend the concept of Community to include all the species of life with which we share the planet. We must foster a reverence for all life, even that which we are forced to control, and we must, as Leopold put it—'Quit thinking about decent land use as solely an economic problem, but examine each question in terms of what is ethically and aesthetically right, as well as what is economically expedient. A thing is right when it tends to preserve the integrity, stability and beauty of the biotic community. It is wrong when it tends otherwise.'

That quotation expresses what I believe should be our guidelines.

To waste, to destroy our natural resources,
    to skin and exhaust the land
instead of using it so as to increase its usefulness,
will result in the undermining in the days of our children
the very prosperity which we ought right
to hand down to them amplified and developed.

—THEODORE ROOSEVELT

Those who contemplate the beauty of the earth
find reserves of strength that will endure
as long as life lasts.

—RACHEL CARSON

Every natural effect has a spiritual cause.

—WILLIAM BLAKE

This Compost

WALT WHITMAN

Something startles me where I thought I was safest,
I withdrew from the still woods I loved,
I will not go now on the pastures to walk,
I will not strip the clothes from my body to meet my lover the sea,
I will not touch my flesh to the earth as to other flesh to renew me.

O how can it be that the ground itself does not sicken?
How can you be alive you growths of spring?
How can you furnish health you blood of herbs, roots, orchards, grain?
Are they not continually putting distemper'd corpses within you?
Is not every continent work'd over and over with sour dead?

Where have you disposed of their carcasses?
Those drunkards and gluttons of so many generations?
Where have you drawn off all the foul liquid and meat?
I do not see any of it upon you to-day, or perhaps I am deceive'd.
I will run a furrow with my plough, I will press my spade through
    the sod and turn it up underneath.
I am sure I shall expose some of the foul meat.

Behold this compost! Behold it well!
Perhaps every mite has once form'd part of a sick person
    —yet behold!
The grass of spring covers the prairies,
The bean bursts noiselessly through the mould in the garden,
The delicate spear of the onion pierces upward,
The apple-buds cluster together on the apple-branches,

The resurrection of the wheat appears with pale visage out of its
    graves,
The tinge awakes over the will-tree and the mulberry-tree,
The he-birds carol mornings and evenings while the she-birds sit on
    their nests,
The young of poultry break through the hatch'd eggs,
The new-born of animals appear, the calf is dropt from
    the cow, the colt from the mare,
Out of its little hill faithfully rise the potato's dark green leaves,
Out of its hill rises the yellow maize-stalk, the lilacs bloom in the
    dooryards,
The summer growth is innocent and disdainful above all those
    strata of sour dead.

What chemistry?
That the winds are really not infectious,
That this is no cheat, this transparent green-wash of the sea which
    is so amorous after me,
That it is safe to allow it to lick my naked body all over with its
    tongues,
That it will not endanger me with the fevers that have deposited
    themselves in it,
That all is clean forever and forever,
That the cool drink from the well tastes so good,
That blackberries are so flavorous and juicy,
That the fruits of the apple-orchard and the orange-orchard, the
    melons, grapes, peaches, plums, will none of them poison me,
That when I recline on the grass I do not catch any disease,
Though probably every spear of grass rises out of what was once a
    catching disease.

Now I am terrified at the Earth, it is that calm and patient,
It grows such sweet things out of such corruptions,
It turns harmless and stainless on its axis, with such
endless successions of diseas'd corpses,
It distills such exquisite winds out of such infused fetor,
It renews with such unwitting looks its prodigal, annual,
    sumptuous crops,
It gives such divine materials to men, and accepts such leavings
    from them at last.

"But there is a principle or quality in the [native] diets which is absent from, or deficient in, the food of our people today...the food is, for the most part, fresh from its source little altered by preparation and complete; and that in the case of those based on agriculture, the natural cycle animal and vegetable—soil—plant—food—man—waste is complete."

"Though we bear no direct responsibility for such problems, yet the better manuring of the homeland so as to bring an ample succession of fresh food crops to the tables of our people, the arrest of the present exhaustion of the soil and the restoration and permanent maintenance of its fertility concern us very closely. For nutrition and the quality of food are the paramount factors in fitness. No health campaign can succeed unless the materials of which the bodies are built are sound. At present they are not."

SIGNED BY 600 BRITISH PHYSICIANS CIRCA EARLY 1900'S
EXCERPTS OF "THE MEDICAL TESTAMENT"

Agriculture, N. [from L. *ager*, field, earth, soil,
and *cultura*, cultivate, care]

The Latin roots of 'agriculture' suggest it to mean
the improvement, refinement and development of the land,
the fields and the earth by study, training and education.

Its usage has long been associated
with the patience and care of *husbandry*.

Organic food consumption
is ecological altruism.

—EDITOR

Why I Consume Organic Food

Dana Pratt, M.S.

Around the world consumers are beginning to take a hard look at their lifestyle practices and the foods they eat. Like many others, I have come to the realization that my health and that of my family is something I can actively protect. One important component of my plan to strive toward optimal health is to provide organic foods at my table as much as possible. There are many reasons for this decision including: common sense, peace of mind, support for reasonable agricultural practices, avoidance of harmful substances, and the love of gardening. This essay will examine each of these reasons more carefully.

Eating wholesome, responsibly-raised foodstuffs is what mankind has done as a natural, common sense approach to providing sustenance throughout the centuries—until ours, that is. In the past, all foods were organic, family-raised products, or at least purchased from local farms or sold at public markets. Historically, all peoples could enjoy fresh fruits and vegetables without questioning their origin and quality. In our modern world, however, such a naive trust of 'store-bought' foods is neither healthy nor wise. As an illustration of the dramatic change in food production, consider the words of Robert Oelhaf in his book entitled *Organic Agriculture*:

> Until the last few decades, eggs had been produced in the same manner for generations. A few dozen or perhaps a couple of hundred chickens were kept in a henhouse on a farm, which also raised a variety of other foodstuffs. The chickens scratched in the dirt, ate bugs and worms, were fertilized by the roosters, and ate feed raised by the farmer. In the fields, weeds were controlled by cultivation; insect and other pests by crop rotation, planting time and other traditional measures. There was some

for the bugs and some for the farmers. The eggs were collected, handled, and packed by hand....

Overwhelmingly, however, modern eggs are produced in large "egg factories" housing thousands or even millions of birds. The system is totally mechanized, with conveyer belts providing food in carefully controlled quantities. Mixed with the feed are antibiotics to speed growth and prevent disease. The individual cages, averaging about one-third of a square foot per hen, provide little room for exercise. Twice during their one-year lives, hens are debeaked—a painful operation into the quick of the beak— to prevent the cannibalism that would result from overcrowding.[2]

Mr. Oelhaf's horrible tale goes on, but this excerpt is sufficiently convincing to indicate that organically-raised foods are the best choice in our generation. I do not want to feed my family second-hand antibiotics, hormones, pesticides, herbicides and all the other toxins in the foods found on the grocer's shelves. In order to avoid these invisible pollutants and to ensure the health of the foods I eat and serve, the old-fashioned simplicity of eating organically raised foods gives me peace of mind.

My family happens to live on a farm and we are able to raise eggs in the hen-scratch approach mentioned above. However, for the most part, organic foods are not as easy to come by as they were in years gone by. Unless one lives in a major metropolitan area, organic foods are often difficult to locate and almost invariably more expensive than their commercial counterparts. While it would be much easier to keep on the blinders and succumb to the ease of purchasing commercially processed foods, it is not something I can do with a clear conscience. When I read information stating; "In 1989, a report sponsored by the Natural Resources Defense Council, Washington DC., estimated that at least 17% of preschool children were exposed to neurotoxic pesticides from fruits and vegetables alone at levels far above those described as safe by the Federal Government,"[3] I am determined to do my best to protect my family. The extra trouble it takes to purchase or grow my own organic foods is worth it because I consider it an investment in my family. It is a wise investment, because its profit shows itself in our current health and well-being, and even in the health of future generations. To me, our health is far more valuable than the nice wardrobe, the fancy car, the extravagant vacation or the bigger house. Similarly, it is a tradeoff in preventive maintenance since the extra money I spend on healthier foods will lead to fewer medical bills, both now and in the future.

I eat organic foods because there are no chemicals used in growing or processing, consequently the foods can be trusted to be safe, nutritious, and unadulterated.

Only a few years ago, you didn't have to worry about weed killer residues in food, because no one used weed killers. Only a few years ago, you could eat a ham without wondering what was used to cure it. But now you know that your ham probably contains calgon, the same water-softening chemical you use in your laundry. There is a chemical to make ice cream hold its shape as it melts. There are hundreds of different chemicals to kill insects and to cure plant diseases, some of them so poisonous that only one drop on your skin is enough to cause serious illness and even death.[4]

In our modern age of a polluted earth—land, water and air—it just makes sense to give my family the best advantage and not add to the pollutants their bodies must cope with by feeding them foods with chemical residues.

As an avid gardener and a mother of two young boys, I would also never want my family to miss the marvelous experiences involved with growing and preserving our own foods. We have had so many joyful times choosing varieties of plants for "this year's garden," planting the tiny seeds, nurturing their growth, inspecting the bugs attracted to our garden, and, of course, reaping our bounty. What could be more satisfying or delicious than picking fresh strawberries for our morning oatmeal, or munching cherry tomatoes while we work or play in the yard? We also appreciate the responsibility we have as parents to raise a generation of children who love the soil and the wholesome foods that can be homegrown in their own backyards. I also find a great sense of accomplishment and comfort in a cupboard full of organic home-canned fruits, vegetables, sauces, and jams that we store against the coming winter as though we were squirrels preparing for the cold days ahead.

Another benefit to organic gardening is the fact that there are so many wonderful varieties of fruits and vegetables that never appear on the a grocery shelf and yet can easily be grown in a garden. These foods include many heirloom varieties and gourmet specialties. In *The Basic Book of Organically Grown Foods*, we find support for the advantages of selecting your own foods.

When you buy tomatoes in the store, you are getting the fruit of a plant that meets the farmer's requirements but not necessarily yours. The same could be said of almost every fruit, vegetable or grain. When a farmer grows tomatoes, for example, he wants plants whose fruit will ripen in unison, be easy to pick, stand up under shipment and yield the maximum number of bushels or tons per acre. Your wishes as a consumer are observed only so long as they don't conflict with his production problems. But when you grow tomatoes in your own garden, you can pick the variety that fully meets your needs. If you want high vitamin C content you can grow DOUBLERICH or HIGH-C tomatoes. If you want plenty of vitamin A you can select CARO-RED.[5]

Chocolate-colored peppers, Easter egg radishes, and baby vegetables are just a few of the many fun and nutritious varieties of produce we have raised in our gardens. Organically raised foods seem to taste so much better and fresher too, especially if they are the long-anticipated fruit of our own labor. Therefore, I eat organic foods because it is both enjoyable and educational for my family to plant and maintain a garden bursting with a wide variety of wholesome foods that have never been touched by a fertilizer or a pesticide, and yet which look and taste much better than anything available in stores.

I also believe organically-raised foods are superior in nutrient density to non-organic products since they are grown on more fertile soil than the commercial crops.

Humus-rich soil improves the food value of plants by providing them with all the nutrients they need in the proper balance. Balance is the key word. When artificial fertilizers are used, the plants' roots are often saturated with an abundance of one nutrient, making it difficult for them to pick up others they need just as much. Since artificial fertilizers present their food in soluble form, the plant can't be selective and you can almost say it is forced to use whatever is given to it.[6]

The natural feeding of crops and crop rotation employed in organic farming produces a better supply of nutrients in the final product. This is the reason that there is no comparison between a store-bought tomato (especially in the winter!) and a home-grown tomato.

I eat commercially-raised organic food because I want to support the growing trend in this country and around the world to propagate foods that have been grown without the use of chemical fertilizers, pesticides, herbicides and other artificial treatments. I feel this is a practical way I can voice my desire for further availability and choices in the varieties of organic foods that are accessible on the local level. Apparently, consumer voices such as mine are indeed being heard as the following quotation illustrates:

> Though millions of Americans still remain in the dark regarding organics, the media is finally beginning to shed light on the positive aspects of responsibly grown, wholesome foods. Both *U.S. News and World Report* and *Food and Wine* ran supportive articles on organics in 1995. *National Geographic* ran a 29-page feature in December which said organics are "shaking the very foundations of agribusiness."

Indeed, recent growth of the industry has been tremendous. The organic foods market had sales of $2.8 billion in 1995, an increase of 21.7 percent from 1994. For the sixth year in a row, organic sales have increased by more than 20 percent.[7]

This ever-increasing demand for organic foods is being met in a variety of creative ways. In conducting an Internet computer search under the topic "organic foods," a wide cross-section of these alternatives can be found. In addition to the typical natural food stores with their lines of organically-raised foods, there is a whole array of approaches to connecting the consumer and the farmer. Large supermarket chains are adding or beefing up their natural food sections in response to demand from their customers. All sorts of published materials supporting organic foods are available from cookbooks to travel guides to organic and health food eateries. These types of materials as well as the organic foods themselves, can be ordered via high technology on the Internet using a mere touch of a button. One method which is catching on is for direct ordering of organic foods— a sort of long-distance grocery shopping. Under this method either a boxed sampler assortment, or items specifically chosen by the consumer, of fresh organically-grown seasonal fruit and vegetables can be shipped directly to the consumer's home. Similarly, farmers' markets, "u-pick farms," farm stands and other direct marketing outlets are alive and well—especially in warm-weather states like California and Florida. In other areas, Community Supported Agriculture is available which is operated as a membership club in which the consumer buys produce directly from an organic farm. One such program in San Diego called Little Creek Acres in Valley Center offers classes, demonstrations and an "Adopt-a-Goat" program, all dedicated to sustainable agriculture. The ten-acre farm has "never had a toxic substance applied" and features 80 raised gardening beds, compost piles, seedling greenhouse, farm stand, bees, dairy goats, herbs, alfalfa, orchard with stone-fruits, apples, subtropicals, citrus, avocados, dwarf and full-size trees, grapes and value-added processes such as juicing and solar drying. The public is invited to visit and learn about all aspects of sustainable living.[8]

This is the type of farm and agriculture that I hope to see continue to grow and flourish in our country, and therefore, I support these practices by purchasing foods raised on such farms. I see organic farming as "not a throwback to previous eras, but an alternative modern system of production, which seeks to rely solely on biological processes, to obtain high quality and yields which are often as good as those achieved using conventional techniques."[9] It is a viable method of agriculture which preserves the land as well as preserving the people who eat its fruits.

In conclusion, I eat organic foods for a multitude of positive reasons, ranging from avoiding harmful chemicals to supporting sustainable agricultural practices. Nevertheless, when it is boiled down to basics, I eat organic foods because it makes good sense. In an age which often calls black white and white black, it is comforting to have the peace of mind that I am doing everything within my power to give my family strong and healthy bodies as they face the world each day.

We have not inherited the earth from our fathers;
we are borrowing it from our children.

—LESTER BROWN

Give us better food
when we're a working
for our lives.

—DICKENS

The further we are from a state of nature,
the more we lose our natural tastes.

—ROUSSEAU

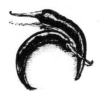

The Culinary Pleasure of Organic Food

Leslie Cerier

I have a love affair with organic cooking that started over twenty years ago. When living in Eastern Kentucky teaching physical education at the university, a colleague brought me to my first natural food store. There, I found shelves of beans and grains I had never seen before. At that time, there were practically no natural food cookbooks.

Like a child, I quizzed the owners of the store. "What is this?" "How do I cook it?" Each visit was an adventure. I bought something new and made up my own recipes.

As a native New Yorker, I soon returned to Manhattan to study creative dance. Often roaming about the city, my quest took me to other neighborhoods and health food stores that stocked organic fruits and vegetables.

Now, living in rural New England, I have found my vocation as an organic gourmet caterer and cookbook author applying creative dance principles to cooking. Using my heart and imagination to prepare meals to support my athletic life-style and satisfy the culinary and health needs of my clients, I have joined a biodynamic farm or "CSA" (community supported farm). Happily, the variety of local organic vegetables and fruits increases each year, as does the distribution of mother earth's bounty from other regions.

The constant change of seasonal ingredients continues to inspire my cooking. Creating new dishes and remaking favorites satisfies the artist in me. Thankfully, organic foods are becoming easier to find in today's local indoor and outdoor markets. There are innumerable fresh, dried and frozen organic foods to easily satisfy moods, cravings and busy schedules.

The bold flavors, colors, and textures of trend-setting organic foods are vital to contemporary life. Popular ethnic flavors, seasonal dishes filled with imagination become a feast for the senses. Cooking with soul-inspiring organic ingredients brings pleasure to the cook and those that eat. Thanks to the organic farmers who attune to the natural rhythms of the seasons as they toil in the fields!

Organic produce looks and tastes fabulous. There is excitement in the garden, on the farm, at the farmer's market, and by the organic produce section of your supermarket. You will find an abundance of choices. It is easy to energize your menus and kitchen with organic foods.

Recently, I taught a cooking class entitled: "Better Beans with Spices." I knew that in class we would prepare a soup with red lentils, ginger and cinnamon. Since it was Fall in my New England town, we would round out the dish with butternut squash and onions.

That morning, as fate would have it, I could not find the recipe. I searched my notebook several times. Open to new possibilities and confident with my skills as an improvisor, I relaxed and let my students guide the recipe.

Magic happens! The soup took on a gorgeous golden color from the melted red lentils and butternut squash. The warm aroma of ginger and cinnamon filled the kitchen. Somehow, however, the dish did not seem complete.

I believe I mentioned something about color, how sometimes it is great to have a dish that is all one color and at other times it is nice to have contrasting colors like natural landscapes. We agreed to add some green. My well-stocked refrigerator included fresh local organic spinach and cilantro. We all agreed to add them to the simmering pot. Quickly we rinsed, chopped, and stirred them into the pot. Instantly, the tender greens wilted. We turned off the heat and got spoons. We tasted it and all agreed it was fabulous. No one wanted to add salt.

By my merely providing an open structure for my students to be spontaneous, they were able to open their hearts and imagination to create a nourishing soup based on local, seasonal organic ingredients.

Here is the recipe. I call it "Sweet Bean Heaven."

Sweet Bean Heaven

Inspired by the richness of flavors and colors of a New England Autumn, this glorious soup is delicious and easy to prepare.

Serves 4-6
Time: 35 minutes

6 cups water
1 cup red lentils, well rinsed
1 cinnamon stick
1 medium-large red or yellow onion, sliced, 1½ cups
1 medium butternut squash, peeled and cubed, 6½ cups
1 inch piece ginger, grated*
Optional: 1 tablespoon dried nettles**
4 cups spinach, rinsed and sliced
1 bunch cilantro, rinsed and sliced, 1 cup
Optional: season to taste with salt

Boil the water while you rinse the lentils. Put the lentils in a stock pot with the cinnamon stick, grated ginger, cubed butternut squash, sliced onions and nettles. Pour in the boiling water. Boil and simmer for at least twenty minutes until the lentils are creamy. Stir in spinach and cilantro. Taste the soup, and season to taste with sea salt, if desired.

* You may peel the ginger if you want. Since I use organic ginger, I do not peel it.

** Nettles are a deeply nourishing wild herb that has a delicate flavor similar to parsley. Dried nettles are sold in many natural food stores.

Variations

Feel free to substitute your favorite quick cooking greens for the spinach. Other possibilities are tat soi and mizuna. Hearty green leafy vegetables such as mustard greens, broccoli, kale and collards are stronger flavored and will not cook down as much. Try adding only one or two cups to preserve the delicate flavor of the soup. They also require a longer cooking time. Simmer the soup an extra five to ten minutes to tenderize and bring out the best in these greens.

The Cinnamon Walnut Coffee Cake

I created this recipe with my daughter Emily, who at the time was in the fourth grade. Another mother brought her eleven year old daughter, Marie, for a private cooking lesson because she wanted to develop a taste for natural foods and health-supportive cooking. Marie loved Drakes' coffee cakes. Drakes are a brand of sugary pastry products sold on the East Coast which contain artificial ingredients. Her mom, Diane, wanted to see if I could invent one with organic ingredients that would meet with her daughter's approval and appease her sweet tooth.

A simple variation to a wonderful and versatile cake recipe produced this coffee cake. Though I had never made a crumb topping before, I believed that mixing a little cinnamon with some ground walnuts and maple syrup would work. Trusting my intuition, I poured some walnuts into a measuring cup. The girls noted the measurement and poured the nuts into the bowl of my food processor, pressed the start button and watched the nuts almost become a paste. I instructed them to add a little maple syrup and cinnamon and once again turn on the food processor and blend them together. After doing this, they tasted it and asked for more maple syrup and cinnamon for a richer flavor.

The girls measured the cake ingredients and mixed them together. They tasted the batter and exclaimed, "Yum." They oiled the cupcake pan and poured in the batter, crumbled the sweetened ground nuts onto each cupcake and put the pan into the preheated oven.

Marie was more than satisfied with the cinnamon walnut cupcakes she helped create. Emily was proud of them, too. Several years have passed. Emily, now a teenager, still loves the recipe I now call "Cinnamon Walnut Coffee Cake." Serving it at business brunches, or yoga and meditation retreats, it pleases both the devout vegetarian and the hungry business communities.

While many coffee cakes rely on high fat sour cream and eggs, this sweet recipe is cholesterol-free and contains no refined sugar. Here is a nice big coffee cake, perfect for brunch, snacks and dessert.

Serves: 12-15
Time: 50 minutes to make and then let it cool before serving

Coffee Cake
3 cups whole wheat pastry flour
1 tablespoon non-aluminum baking powder
⅜ teaspoons sea salt
1 tablespoon cinnamon

½ cup Canola oil
½ cup maple syrup
1½ cups apple juice

Crumb topping
1½ cups walnuts
5 tablespoons maple syrup
2½ teaspoons cinnamon

Preheat the oven to 350 degrees. In a large mixing bowl combine all the cake ingredients. There is no need to sift the flour unless you want to do it. Stir well to blend the ingredients. Take a lick, and adjust the seasonings, if desired. Lightly oil a 9x13x2 inch Pyrex glass pan. Pour in the cake batter.

Grind up the walnuts in a food processor and than add the cinnamon and maple syrup and blend well. Taste the mixture and adjust the flavor, if desired. Crumble the sweetened walnuts onto the cake batter. Bake for 30 minutes, or until an inserted tooth pick comes out dry.

Variations
Add a teaspoon of vanilla to the cake batter and/or the crumb topping.

Grandma's Chicken Soup

My two grandmothers loved to cook. Both were excellent bakers and made wonderful lunches for our family visits with many of their trademark dishes. They made their own cookies, salad dressings, soups— you name it. They loved to fuss for us. Their love went into the pot along with their great intuition.

My grandmother Ethel used to go down to the chicken market on the lower east side of Manhattan. There she would pick out a live chicken for the evening's meal. She had a friendly relationship with the butcher, and he would give her a fair deal and pure food.

These days, you can still get the best meat and poultry by knowing your source. Free range poultry is becoming a popular item. The standard practice of chaining animals and injecting them with harmful hormones and antibiotics is unappealing. Educated consumers question where their food has been before they buy and serve it.

Whether you are a vegetarian or meat eater, the food on your plate contains a life force, a spirit beyond its physical molecules. The way the food is grown, transported to the marketplace and displayed is just the beginning. The mood of the cook, the artistic presentation of the meal, the rhythm of our chewing, and the company we keep during the meal also becomes a part of what we digest.

Luckily, as I mentioned, I belong to a community-supported biodynamic farm. Not only do they grow the tastiest fruits and vegetables, but they also raise pigs and chickens that breath the clean air, drink the pure water and feast on the extra organic vegetables, hay and grains from the farm. These animals live in large fields and have frequent friendly visits by many of the farm members and their children. Their meat is extremely lean from their diet high in greens.

This year I evoked the spirit of my Grandma Ethel as I prepared my first chicken soup in twenty years. I could not resist buying a couple of these chickens since they were so well cared for and fed. Though it is rare for me to eat meat, I enjoyed a bowl of this chicken soup as part of a special holiday dinner.

Feel free to vary the vegetables and add your favorite herbs and spices. I started with a very large chicken, about 5 pounds. Most organic chickens in the store are smaller. That is why I will suggest a range of amounts for vegetables.

1 whole chicken
4 quarts water
1 tablespoon sea salt
1-3 onions, 3 cups chunky cut onions
½–1 pound carrots, "roll" or chunky cut, 2–4 cups
2–4 stalks celery with their leaves, if you have them, 1–4 cups

Cut away as much chicken fat and skin as you can. Rinse the chicken. Put it in a large stock pot with water. Change the water several times until it runs clear, then add 4 quarts of water or just enough to barely cover the chicken. It is okay for the wings and drum-sticks to stick out. Add salt.

Turn the heat on high while you cut up the vegetables. You can use one large carrot, one onion, and two stalks of celery for a small chicken. This recipe is flexible. The slow, long simmering of the chicken makes the soup delicious cooked with one or more quarts of vegetables. It is entirely up to you. Use more vegetables when you have a large chicken. For example, a three pound chicken may require up to five pounds of vegetables.

Add the cut vegetables. Put the lid on the pot. When the water reaches a rolling boil, turn the heat down to a simmer. Flip the chicken over as often as you like, perhaps every 10-15 minutes or even longer. Since the chicken is not fully submerged, flipping it over with tongs insures even cooking. After 1½ to 2 hours, the meat will easily fall off the bones as you turn the chicken. The wings and drum sticks will fall off with a gentle push with a long spoon. The chicken is now fully submerged in soup. Simmer the soup a full two hours for a very savory flavor. Then you can easily pick and poke the skin off, discard the bones and tear the chicken into bite-sized pieces.

Variations

1. You can chop up and add a fresh bunch of dill at the end of cooking the soup.
2. You can simmer the soup with an astragalus stick, which boosts the immune system. Discard it before you serve the soup.
3. You can simmer the soup with garlic and/or ginger
4. You can add turnips and parsnips to the soup.

The romance of organic food begins with a dazzling abundance of color, flavor and nutrition. A daily ritual, cooking is like a game. Mixing and matching seasonal fruits and vegetables with herbs and spices offers us a chance to go around the world without leaving the kitchen. The combinations seem infinite.

Pleasant, memorable meals with the conversation and laughter of family and friends inspire organic cooking. Culinary pleasure comes to us when we cast our spell on food, magically transforming it into light and delectable appetizers, savory entrees, creamy dressings, refreshing salads, spicy side dishes, and sweet desserts. We may view cooking as a means to an end or our sincere expression of gratitude for the earth's bounty.

Finding pleasure in touching, smelling, and tasting healthy organic foods unites us with the effort and work of many beings and forces: farmers, grocers, truckers, the sun, the rain, and mother earth. As we share in this sensual splendor, we say yes to life. Connecting to the source, organic farms and gardens bring us meals that warm the heart, feed the soul and honor the earth.

A garden grown as one should be,
without chemical sprays or fertilizers,
will produce vegetables which are superior
in taste and quality.

—SAMUEL R. OGDEN

One cannot think well, love well,
sleep well, if one has not dined well.

—VIRGINIA WOOLF

Seeing is deceiving.
It's eating that's believing.

—JAMES THURBER

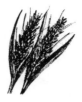

My Life in Organics

FRANK FORD

Deaf Smith County

The Ford Farm was located in Deaf Smith County which many authories consider to have the richest topsoil in the country.

Erastus Smith was deaf from his youth. His parents moved from New York, where he was born, to Mississippi when he was young. In his early twenties, he left his comfortable home and wealthy background to go to the frontier of Texas. He married a beautiful woman named Guadalupe Ruiz Duran, and they had several children together.

In the mid 1830's, war broke out between Santa Anna, the Emperor of Mexico, and the settlers from various Eastern states. In 1836, "Deaf" Smith tried to enter his home village of San Antonio, and General Cos, a brother-in-law to Santa Anna, ordered his pickets to shoot at him. Until then, he had no quarrel with anyone; afterwards, he joined Gen. Sam Houston's army in the final battle for Texas independence. At age 48, he became the foremost hero at San Jacinto. He was a scout with keen eyes, and on the day of the battle, he rode eight miles, chopping down a bridge to cut off the escape for Santa Anna's army. He then rode back and fought hand-to-hand that afternoon. He later became a captain in the Texas Rangers shortly before his death in his early fifties.

Captain Smith was a poet and a man of great character. Deaf Smith County was named after him, located in the Southwest corner of the Texas Panhandle.

Wheat Planting 1974

Between 1947 and 1975, my farming day started at 4 am and continued until it was too dark to see. The crops I raised included wheat, rye, grain, sorghum, feed and hay.

During wheat planting in the fall of 1974, I had a week to remember. I hadn't intended to put in 123 hours that week, but a full moon early on and the fragrance of the rich soil kept me going until midnight each night. On Thursday, I felt so excited about how well things were going that I slept only an hour under the 930 Case tractor. In six days, I seeded 1,200 acres of organic wheat without a single equipment break, and no other person in the fields. The two old Van Brunt drills had to be filled with 2,500 lbs. of seed every four hours. There was diesel fueling every seven hours, and 80 grease points every five hours. While the fuel flowed into the tractor I would grab a half dozen pears off the organic pear trees. Otherwise, all I ate that week was a handful of wheat from the drill each time I checked them. Needless to say, it wasn't treated seed.

That crop turned out 30 bushels per acre in late June 1975. The Llano Estacado, which occupies most of the Western Half of the Texas Panhandle, is fertile country.

Composting

We are blessed to have three or four top-quality composters in the area. The techniques were pioneered by people who were committed to returning feed lot manure to the soil. The heat of the compost killed the seeds of most weeds before they could grow. Inoculation further increased the micro-life of the soil.

Pest Control

With a healthy soil, I was never once troubled by soil or plant disease. The beneficial insects (ladybugs, lacewing flies and tiny braconid wasps) seemed to greatly appreciate the fact that no chemical sprays were used against their natural realm.

In 27 years of organic wheat farming, the ladybugs and lacewing fly larvae never once failed to come to the rescue in the warm Spring months when greenbug and brown mite infestations would threaten the winter wheat crop as it began to grow. The adult ladybugs were hungry, but the ½" long larvae, as they hatched from gold eggs, which were laid in clusters under the dry "cowchips," and which resembled orange and black gila monsters, were voracious. The lacewing larvae, a little longer than the ladybug larvae and black and white in color, were similarly helpful.

Soil and Grain Testing

I had done extensive tests with soil amendments to increase the God-given natural fertility of our three-foot deep clay-loam topsoil. I had used compost from our abundant sources, gypsum (calcium sulfate) and some of the soft coal humates that had triggered better earthworm activity on the organic farms of the Midwest. I even tried some bat guano from the caves of Central Texas.

In order to measure the results, I had soil tests run with Brookside Laboratories. After harvest, tests were run on both the trace mineral content of the grain, the test weight, and the protein. Protein ran above 17% in that special year of 1972, and the test weight was an unbelievable 66 lbs. per bushel.* Climactic and soil conditions never again brought such remarkable results, but there is little doubt that the claims of A.W. Erickson, a very prominent soil scientist from Minnesota, that we had the best soil in the U.S. had merit. He did his studies in the 1930s and 1940s and that, along with a READER'S DIGEST article in 1947 about the natural fluorides and good calcium and magnesium in our underground water table in the area, were the basis for my enterprise.

Arrowhead Mills

It was an overwhelming desire to create a larger market for organically-grown wheat that caused me to start Arrowhead Mills in 1960. I have always believed in small business and in the quality that comes from people who care.

The early years were difficult ones. I would work eighteen-hour days, dividing my time between an old LA Case tractor and a $400 pickup truck which I used to haul cases of organic stone-ground wheat

---

*Editor's note: the typical protein content of winter wheat is about 12%, and the standard bushel weight is around 60 lbs.

and cornmeal to local food stores. Local, in this case, meant traveling up to 150 miles to make a delivery. On a good day, sales were $40-$50.

My office was an old rail-car with a shed attached to it. I built four grain bins with hampered bottoms, hammering through solid rock to dig a central boot pit. A 1,000 square foot warehouse was constructed to serve the lone thirty-inch Meadows grain mill.

I invested in a truck which cost $450 and had 500,000 miles on it. But it would generally reach the bakery, 100 miles away, which I had garnered as an account. And the business began to grow. Nevertheless, I could not pay myself salary for seven of the first ten years.

By 1970, Arrowhead Mills had become viable, and our product line, that now included pinto beans and soybeans, was being motor-freighted from coast to coast. However, freight costs were high, damaged bags were common, and I saw the need to develop a distribution system which allowed for the delivery of full truckload quantities to key destinations in major cities.

There were other visionaries at this time who saw this same need, and together, we began to "plot" the natural food revolution. Out of this strategic planning came the vast network of distributors and stores which now has become one of the fastest-growing industries in our nation.

What was the spirit and purpose of this revolution? It was originally a return to the soil and the land which had been devastated by the blitz of high-nitrate fertilizers and chemical pesticides. More specifically, it was a reaction to the destruction of the micro-life and tilth in the soil and the pollution of our air and water as well as the cells of all living creatures.

At the food chain level, it was evident to many that the heavy doses of innumerable coloring agents, preservatives and taste enhancers, including large doses of salt, were having a severe negative effect on the health of our citizens. While the cost of our country's health care was dramatically rising, the quality of its people's actual health was in a dramatic decline.

The understanding of these dangerous trends led many young people to make a stand for the environment and for personal health nearly a quarter of a century ago. Arrowhead Mills was a part of this counter-movement, the organic revolution, which is still gaining momentum today.

Publicity/Deaf Smith Cookbook

Many T.V. and print media stories were done about my farm in the Western part of Deaf Smith County in the 1970s and early 80s. In one of these, P.M. Magazine sent a four-person crew from N.Y., and that came at a time when the infestation of "bad bugs" was a heavy one indeed. They got so excited in seeing the "good guys" cleaning up on the wee "black hat villains" that they actually were jumping with joy as their zoom lenses gave then a front row seat on the drama of nature at work.

John Deere did two stories, one on my terracing, and one on the use of balance of nature in insect control. CBN did a T.V. special, and the "New York Times" not only did a large story in their own paper, but syndicated it all over the U.S. That story led to several cookbook offers, one which led to the DEAF SMITH COOKBOOK which sold roughly 350,000 copies. Many people have said that this book was the foundation of what became an expanding library of good natural food cookbooks in their kitchens. THE SIMPLER LIFE COOKBOOK, which my wife and I wrote as an off-spring, then sold 650,000 copies, but it was printed in a dime-novel format and not the quality hardback of its predecessor.

Organic Gardening

As an organic gardener during my farming days and afterward, I was successful in raising about 30 types of vegetables; and pears, peaches, and apricots in a rather sizable orchard. The decision I made as a young man to farm organically was a joy. The air was purer, and the soil often smelled so good as the lively micro-life converted atmospheric nitrogen into useable plant food. The extensive terraces on the farm let little water escape, and there was little soil erosion. It is now a better place than it was.

Last year (1996), my wife and I had a 1,600 sq. ft. organic garden. Five tons of compost were incorporated, and the rains came in a manner that made watering requirements minimal. We had abundant black-eyed peas, green beans, lima beans, squash, peppers, tomatoes, beets, Swiss chard, cucumbers, cantaloupes, watermelons, garlic, parsley, okra and giant sunflowers. We had one okra plant that liked our soil fertility so well it grew 12 feet tall. We also had 17 varieties of flowers. On none of these were any pesticides used, though I did have to spray soapy water to curtail squashbugs. If I had waited until mid-July to plant the three varieties of squash, I think we would have missed the squashbug cycle. They are pernicious little buggers.

Just this morning in mid-April, of 1997, we bought some strawberries and brought some in from our own organic garden. The taste is definitely superior of the organically-grown strawberries, and with tomatoes and many other vegetables, it is even more so. For those who don't have a garden plot, I would highly recommend that a few pots with good potting soil will provide taste and pleasure for the entire family. It has always been a thrill for me to see things grow, and the smell of the good earth, rather than the unhealthy and unpleasant smell of chemicals so prevalent in many lawn and garden outlets, is magnificent.

Mealtime

A typical evening meal when I was on the farm (after a whole grain breakfast and a light lunch as I generally kept going during daylight) would be:

- A soybean-based casserole
- Whole wheat rolls
- Two or three vegetables dishes, depending on season
- A salad from the garden (raw foods especially need to be organically grown)
- Herb tea

Although I am now retired from organic farming and marketing, I continue to eat, almost exclusively, organic foods.

I begin the day with a piece of fruit and then go for an hour swim or walk. I must admit that I have not been able to shake my "up at 4 am" farming habit, so this occurs earlier than most people would think sensible. After the sunrise, I enjoy a breakfast of whole grain cereal, usually mixed from two or three varieties, with a banana and soy milk. Lots of fresh vegetables form the basis of my other two meals which are also heavy with soy products and whole grains. I often enjoy fresh fruit as a between-meal snack.

I will admit to being a believer in supplements, including a raw green supplement and vitamin C when I get up at night and some

Omega 3 oil with the fruit first thing in the morning. A good multi-vitamin-mineral supplementation and generous use of herbs can, I believe, give most people a needed margin against today's fast pace.

Dr. Roger J. Williams

I was privileged to know and learn from Dr. Roger J. Williams, a great man of science, and to spend many hours with him in his laboratory in Austin, Texas. Dr. Williams was a bio-chemist who wrote many books on health and nutrition and was a major force in encouraging medical schools to teach nutrition as a science and as a form of preventative medicine. He was the only biochemist who served as president of The American Chemical Society, and he remained active and productive into his nineties.

Dr. Williams knew and taught that "we are all extraordinary" and greatly influenced me in this respect. I believe that we are all unique individuals and our bodies are our temples. Eating organic food can help keep our bodies cleansed and our lives full and vibrant.

Philosophy of Sustainability

It has been over 17 years since Alvin Toffler wrote *The Third Wave and the Coming of the Electronic Age.* We are certainly in the midst of that wave now, and while it creates so many new opportunities and improves the quality of life for millions of us, the increasingly rapid pace of life signals a challenge as well.

We need a quiet place where we can watch nature's timeless miracles. This place can be a basepoint of tranquillity and pleasure for those who take the time to integrate it into their daily lives.

An organic garden can be a part of this "organic" lifestyle. The word that I have tried to use most often, in hundreds of radio and T.V. appearances and in hundreds of lectures relating to my chosen profession, is "sustainability." Are we, as individuals and as a society, operating in a sustainable manner?

Each of us, if we are seeking that standard in our lives, has to answer that question in our own way. Yet it is a high standard and one worthy of the seeking.

Osiris and Isis were at one time induced
to descend to the earth to bestow gifts
and blessings on its inhabitants.
Isis showed them first the use of wheat and barley,
and Osiris made the instruments of agriculture
and taught men the use of them,
as well as how to harness the ox to the plow.

—BULLFINCH'S MYTHOLOGY

I know of no pursuit in which more real and important services
can be rendered to any country than by improving its agriculture.

—GEORGE WASHINGTON

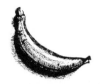

Organic Agriculture and the World Food Supply[1]

FREDERICK KIRSCHENMANN, PH.D.

In 1798 Thomas Malthus, an English clergyman and political economist, published a treatise entitled Essay on the Principle of Population that riveted the world's attention, for the first time, on the "problem" of human population growth. Malthus argued that population growth was bound to outstrip food production since unchecked human population would grow geometrically while the food supply could, at best, only grow arithmetically.

Malthus' powerful thesis has been the basis for justifying numerous social doctrines ever since—everything from the "survival of the fittest" to the "green revolution." During the last decade the Malthusian thesis has been revived to justify intensive, industrial agriculture technologies, including genetic engineering. The argument goes something like this: if we don't use these technologies, even though there may be some risk in doing so, and even though there may be some harm to the environment, millions of people will starve to death.

This way of posing the argument has turned the issue into a moral plea. For example, in his essay in praise of Norman Borlaug, published in the January, 1997 issue of The Atlantic Monthly magazine, Gregg Easterbrook blames all those who oppose green revolution technologies for the starvation of people in Africa. Borlaug was, of course, the agronomist who developed the high-yielding grain varieties (and the input-intensive technologies required to produce those yields) ushering in the new era of industrial agriculture. The moral defense of Easterbrook's essay is clear. Those who oppose high-input agriculture will have starving millions on their conscience (Easterbrook, 1996)!

Posing the problem this way makes it appear that the Malthusian dilemma can be solved by simply inventing the technologies to continue producing enough food to stay ahead of population growth.

Aside from the fact that many technology experts are now questioning whether additional technologies can increase yields, there are several more fundamental misapprehensions with this oversimplification of the problem.

First, human population cannot continue to grow at anything like its present rate even if we can invent the technologies to feed everyone. Present levels of human population are already causing a serious imbalance relative to the millions of other species with whom we co-evolved. This imbalance will increasingly disrupt and deteriorate our ecosystems, and it is that disruption and deterioration (and the subsequent loss of ecosystem services vital to food production) which threatens the long term food supply of the human species.

Since many of the intensive, industrial agriculture technologies being proposed as the solution to food shortage problems are known to dramatically increase ecological disruption and deterioration, intensifying them will only further threaten the ability of future generations to feed themselves. So even if such technologies are able to increase the yields of a few crop varieties for the short term, it is doubtful that they will alleviate the problem of hunger in the long term.

Second, the assumption that technology alone must be credited with increasing our food supplies is seriously flawed. In his provocative study, The Genesis Strategy, world renowned climatologist, Stephen Schneider demonstrated that both increased crop yields and low yield variability are due at least as much to weather as to technology (Schneider, 1976). I suppose any farmer could have told him that.

Because weather is such a significant factor in our capacity to produce high yields, Schneider argues that, if we want to keep the world fed, we need to implement the strategy of the biblical Joseph who urged Egypt to store part of the abundance of the seven good years to assure themselves food for the seven bad years. This has more to do with how we manage our food supply than it does with the technologies we use to produce it.

But pointing out the wisdom of grain storage to see us through periods of weather-related disasters is only a small part of Schneider's premise. He points out how small changes in atmospheric conditions can cause major changes in weather patterns. That should remind us how important it is for us to use farming practices that do not contribute to the destabilization of delicately balanced atmospheric conditions.

We know, for example, that global warming could radically disrupt earth's weather patterns, causing significant weather fluctuations and an increase in violent storms. And those changes can dramatically change our ability to produce food. So how we respond to the threat of global warming and the technologies that cause it may be more important for an adequate food supply than inventing new technologies that increase food production.

Third, posing the problem of adequate food supplies exclusively in terms of intensive agricultural technologies to increase crop production misinterprets the true nature of our food supply. 60% of the world's population today depends on fish and seafood for 40% of its annual protein (Hewitt and Smith, 1995). According to some reports "insects provide the major source of protein to roughly 60% of the world's population" (Spindler and Schultz, 1996:65). These, and other vital food sources are often ignored in the "feeding the world" debate.

In fact, there is a tendency to equate grain yields with food production. Easterbrook, for example, credits Norman Borlaug with saving "more lives than any other person who ever lived" because Borlaug increased grain yields of a few crops two and three-fold (Easterbrook, 1996). However, it is well known that the very technologies that accomplished the increased grain yields have seriously damaged seafood ecologies. So, an important question has to be asked. Do we really increase food production when we increase wheat and rice yields at the expense of seafood?

There are, in fact, serious doubts as to whether or not the green revolution methods actually produce more food despite producing higher yields of a few crops. In her well-documented book, The Violence of the Green Revolution, Vandana Shiva points out numerous problems with the Green Revolution in India. She points out, for example, that while the Green Revolution "miracle seeds" were more responsive to chemical fertilizer and irrigation inputs, their overall performance was inferior to the indigenous seeds selected and bred by India's farmers for centuries (Shiva 1991:61f). In fact, Shiva argues that when all factors are taken into account India's food security was probably diminished, rather than enhanced, by the Green Revolution.

Furthermore, India experienced detrimental side effects from the green revolution agriculture in India. According to a Science magazine article, people in various regions of India have, for some time, been suffering from strange outbreaks of arsenic poisoning. The article points out that the poisoning was finally traced to increased irrigation. Dramatic increases in irrigation became necessary to produce the increased wheat yields of the high-yielding varieties. It seems that arsenic is naturally present in the soil, and as long as India's farmers only used the limited irrigation required by their own drought-resistant seeds, the arsenic posed no problem to human or animal health. However, the dramatic increase of irrigation required by the high response seeds of the Green Revolution concentrated the arsenic and caused it to leach into the groundwater. Even if industrial agriculture increased grain production in India, it did so (in some locations) at the expense of human health (Bagla and Kaiser, 1996).

Fourth, posing the food/population problem solely in terms of technology's ability to increase grain production ignores the role which animals play in our food system. Much of our capacity to feed the world is wasted because we feed most of our grain protein to animals instead of feeding it directly to humans. However, it does not follow that we should therefore eliminate animals from the food system altogether, as some have argued (Rifkin, 1992). Ruminant animals are the only creatures capable of transforming grass into protein that can be digested by humans. Consequently, if it weren't for animals, over a billion acres in the U.S. alone could not be used for human food. That acreage is unsuitable for crop production. Furthermore, without animals many other feed stuffs not suitable for human consumption (such as crop residues, weather damaged grain, garbage, etc.) could not be turned into protein for humans. If it weren't for animals those waste materials would probably end up in landfills instead of being converted to proteins to feed humans.

Animals not only play a key role in keeping the world fed (especially in Third world countries), they are an important ingredient in mirroring and maintaining the ecological health of local ecosystems. However, in industrial agriculture, animals are unnecessarily fed huge quantities of grain that could otherwise be fed directly to humans. The principle reason for feeding large quantities of grain to animals is that industrial agriculture has concentrated animals in large feed-lots and hog and poultry barns. This concentration of animals makes it inefficient to feed animals forages, crop residues, and wild produc-tion. Transportation costs alone dictate that protein fed to animals must be in concentrated form. Consequently in feedlots, feed rations for animals now consist of up to 90% grain.

Fifth, there are other ecologically related problems that threaten our food supply which cannot be overcome with industrial technolo-gies. For example, many scientists now worry that the combination of increased world trade and intensive mono-cropping agriculture could cause serious food production disruptions. Dramatic increases in world trade augment the likelihood that "invader species" will hitchhike to new ecosystems in which they did not evolve (Baskin, 1996). Many of these species, especially microbial and insect species, could experience population explosions in ecologies where they did not evolve with natural predators—like the explosion of the rabbit population in Australia. Such pest outbreaks could drastically reduce crop production.

At the same time that world trade increases the likelihood of in-vader species, many of the ecosystems into which those species will be introduced are now made much more vulnerable by the special-ization of industrial agriculture. Industrial agriculture now depends on only 15 varieties of plant species world-wide for 90 percent of the calories used to feed the world (Soule,1990). The combination of this dramatic specialization of agriculture (resulting in very brittle eco-systems) and the dramatic increase in the potential for invader spe-cies into those brittle ecologies is a prescription for food supply di-saster. The 19th century Irish potato blight and the corn leaf blight of the 1960's should serve as reminders of how vulnerable genetically uniform cropping systems can be.

It is interesting to note (contrary to Easterbrook's vision for saving Africa from starvation) that the National Research Council has now concluded that it may be necessary for Africa to return to the more than 2,000 indigenous species of grains, fruits, vegetables and roots to reduce the continent's vulnerability to food shortages (NRC, 1996). That advice may become especially critical if local ecosystems, domi-nated by monoculture agriculture, are disrupted by invader species.

The destabilization that may be caused by invader species through increased world trade could be further exacerbated by the simultaneous introduction of novel, genetically engineered organisms, which some scientists have referred to as "aliens with a capital 'A'" (Baskin, 1996). Some scientists have, in fact, suggested that the ecological risks of introducing genetically engineered organisms "are similar in some ways to those of introductions of non-native organisms into new environments" (Rissler and Mellon, 1996; Snow and Palma, 1997).

Finally, the assumption that adequate food supplies can be made available to feed an expanding population with industrial technologies ignores the fact that hunger often has more to do with politics than with production. Ten years ago in a report to the Bruntland Commission the issue of food and population was put into proper perspective. The report said that "The problem is not one of global food production being outstripped by population . . . The problem has three aspects: where the food is being produced, by whom, and who can command it" (Food 2000, 1987).

Reducing the problem of hunger to inadequate production is simply to misconstrue the problem, either inadvertently (due to a lack of understanding) or purposefully (in an attempt to protect vested interests). The fact that there are 800 million starving people on the planet today when we clearly still have the capacity to feed everyone, makes it abundantly clear that hunger today is not a production problem!

At the last World Food Summit a gathering of over 1200 NGO's (non-governmental organizations) put their finger on the problem of food shortages. While the official delegates (heads of state, presidents, prime ministers and ministers of agriculture) proposed that the solution to the problem of world hunger could be achieved through trade liberalization and free market initiatives, the NGO's (represented by farmers, food security activists and anti-hunger advocates) rejected market-driven food security in favor of "farmer and community-driven food security." The title of the NGO's statement revealed their understanding of the nature of the hunger problem: "Profit For Few Or Food For All: Food Sovereignty and Security to Eliminate the Globalization of Hunger."

The contradiction in the official summit position lies in the fact that the global food market responds to money, but most of the 800 million who are starving have no economic power. One does not have to go to Africa to see this problem at work. One need only go to the poor neighborhoods (both rural and urban) in the United States where 12 million children go to bed hungry every night. The problem is indeed one of where the food is produced, by whom and who commands it.

Who "commands the food," of course, has to do with power, not production. Power is perhaps also the reason that we still talk about this subject in terms of "feeding the world," rather than keeping the world fed. "Feeding the world" suggests that someone will take responsibility for feeding someone else, and therefore make them dependent. Under those terms, there can be no food security. "Keeping the world fed" suggests that people will be empowered to feed themselves. And such empowerment is essential to long-term food security.

Given this perspective on the Malthusian dilemma, how does organic agriculture (often castigated by industrial agriculture proponents as an agriculture that would consign half the world to starvation) measure up to the problem?

Organic agriculture attempts to farm in harmony with nature. It seeks to fit agriculture into nature, rather than controlling or dominating nature. Accordingly, while organic agriculture (like any farming activity) disrupts nature, it does so by mimicking and mirroring nature and therefore causes minimum deterioration of the ecosystems in which it is practiced. As organic systems become more elegant ecologically, they also can restore, and in some instances enhance natural systems. Gary Nabhan suggests numerous ways in which farming can perform such functions (Nabhan, 1996 & 1997).

Since organic agriculture uses virtually no exogenous inputs, it is less likely to disturb atmospheric conditions. Organic farms, for example, do not release nitrous oxide into the atmosphere. While organic farmers use fossil fuels for traction energy (although a few use horses) and some may use more traction fuel than no-till farmers, studies have indicated that organic farms use much less energy than conventional or no-till farmers when total energy flows are calculated. In fact a North Dakota study which did actual on-farm comparisons revealed that organic farmers used up to 70% less energy (Clancy, 1993).

Proponents of industrial agriculture often charge that organic agriculture would require that more fragile land be brought under cultivation because organic farms experience lower yields. That charge has never been substantiated by independent research. In fact, "in the field" studies have consistently shown that well managed organic farms experience yields that are comparable to those of conventional farms (Clancy, 1993).

Furthermore, since organic agriculture relies on cropping diversity to control weeds and maintain nutrient levels, the risk of crop loss due to inclement weather and pests is minimized. If a farmer is predominantly a wheat farmer, wheat scab disease can wipe out her entire crop (and thereby dramatically reduce the amount of food she produces). If that same farmer raises six or seven different crops in a rotation, the wheat scab disease will only affect a small part of the farm's production and have a minor impact on the total food the farm produces.

But perhaps even more important for future food security is the fact that organic agriculture increases biodiversity. Since organic farmers use diverse cropping systems, they tend to have smaller fields with more field barriers. That increases habitat for wildlife and for predators that help control crop pests. Consequently wildlife is increased on the farm, where most of the land is, and not just in wilderness areas.

Biodiversity is also increased by improved soil quality. Fertile soil is essential for organic farm production since no imported fertilizers are used. Improved soil quality enhances soil microbial life which, in turn, is the first stage of a vibrant food chain that nurtures a healthy biotic community. Quality, organically-nurtured soil is also the "bank" that insures future food security.

However, we should not delude ourselves into believing that the human species can continue to populate itself at anything like its present rate of growth no matter what agriculture systems we use. The human species is part of an intricate biotic community, and therefore we have to maintain some kind of equilibrium with other species in that community if we are to survive with any kind of quality of life. Feeding itself from that community is only one of a very complex set of problems which an overburdening human population poses. Maintaining all of the ecological relationships between diffusely co-evolved species will be absolutely essential to survival.

But organic agriculture, inserted into the current industrial food system infrastructure, will fare no better at feeding the world than industrial agriculture. The NGO's at the World Food Summit had it right—the only kind of food system that can keep the world fed is a "farmer and community-driven food security." It is becoming increasingly clear that apart from this kind of radical restructuring of the food system we will have little success in keeping the world fed. Meeting maximum production goals of a few crops and livestock in a few regions of the world, to be marketed into the global economy, will not keep the world fed.

Following the sentiment of the Bruntland report, many are now concluding that the best way to achieve food security is through local food produced by local people with local control. Such a local food system allows for the evolution of a people/food/land equilibrium based on local culture.

There is substantial evidence to suggest that the best way to achieve such people/food/land equilibrium is through local community-based agriculture, tied to ecologically responsible local land use, rooted in local culture. Helena Norberg-Hodge (1991) provides us with an intriguing example of such a food system in her study of the Ladakh. Despite very scarce resources and extreme climates, the Ladakhi people, living in the desert highlands of the Western Himalayas, are well nourished, usually healthy and free of social and environmental stresses (Kirschenmann, 1997).

The Ladakhi experience corroborates one of the principles for ending hunger outlined by Francis Moore Lappe:

> While slowing population growth in itself cannot end hunger, the very changes necessary to end hunger—the democratization of economic life, especially the empowerment of women—are key to reducing birth rates so that the human population can come into balance with the rest of the natural world (Lappe and Collins, 1986).

We still don't know the capacity of a people in a local ecological neighborhood to feed themselves, once they are empowered to properly use local resources and sound ecological farming systems. Different ecological neighborhoods would have different capacities, depending on local climate, land and sea-based food resources. Exporting surpluses from one foodshed to another could, of course, always continue to be part of the new food system. But, the first priority in the new food system would be food self-sufficiency in every ecological neighborhood. Furthermore, local food systems, tied to local ecological neighborhoods would tend to create people/food/land equilibrium through local culture, as it has among the Ladakh.

This vision of the restructuring of the global food system may seem bizarre in our world of global markets and global competitiveness. But the World Food Summit revealed that very different views on the issue exist. While government and industry representatives officially expressed the notion that global competitiveness and transnational corporations were the answer to food security, 1200 NGO's saw them as the cause of food insecurity.

It is interesting to note that regional foodshed concepts have usually only been endorsed by grass-roots groups and food activists. More recently, the idea is being endorsed by the U.S. Congress in programs like the Community Food Security Act and by researchers in land grant universities. Jack Kloppenburg and his colleagues at the University of Wisconsin, in an article on "Coming Into the Foodshed" (Kloppenburg, et. al., 1996), concluded that regional foodsheds were not only desirable but feasible.

Cornelia Flora at Iowa State University is now suggesting that food and farming systems should model themselves after the new economy rather than the old industrial economy. The old economy was modeled after "Fordism"—mass production of a uniform commodity at a low price. In other words, produce more wheat for less money. The new economy relies on the production of differentiated products produced on a much smaller scale, but designed to be innovative and flexible to meet the fast-changing demands of a discriminating consumer (Flora, 1996). The post-Fordist economy generally shortens supply lines and responds to local markets. It doesn't attempt to compete in the global mass market. This localized, site-specific concept of the economy can also be adapted to empowering local people to feed themselves.

It now turns out that food safety may ultimately also depend on a more diverse, ecologically oriented food system. In her provocative new book, Spoiled: The Dangerous Truth About a Food Chain Gone Haywire, Nicols Fox concludes that "Whenever there is a lack of diversity, when a standardized food product is mass-produced, disease can enter the picture" (Fox, 1997).

Fortunately, the idea of local foodsheds, stocked with a diversity of locally produced foods, is catching on in many local communities, especially among poor neighborhoods. USDA's Community Food Security program has revealed that throughout the United States hundreds of communities are creating new food and farming markets. In many instances organic farmers are linking with community organizations to exchange food for labor, community gardens are linked with local school systems to provide food for poor families and teach kids how to do organic gardening, and local businesses work with non-profit organizations to make food available in communities without grocery stores.

These fledgling enterprises, together with the growing Farmers Markets, direct marketing arrangements and Community Supported Agriculture, are all indications that the global industrial food system is not working for a growing number of people. Accordingly, new food systems, grounded in local culture, sound local ecological management and local control, are likely to make up an increasing portion of the food system of tomorrow.

Making such fundamental shifts in the food system is, however, bound to run into opposition. Since agriculture today is about power, powerful interests will oppose these new initiatives and, of course, continue to claim that only their way can prevent world starvation.

Nevertheless, if organic agriculture remains true to its ecological roots, and reaffirms its vision of a farmer and community-driven food system, it could play a key role in keeping the world fed. International trade could continue to play a secondary role of supplementing such a food system with exotic foods that can't be produced locally, and to meet weather related food shortage emergencies. Such a system could conceivably keep the world fed.

Try producing truly abundant,
naturally blessed food
that serves as a real source of life
and have all the people of the nation
eat a full and wholesome diet. . .

—MASANOBU FUKUOKA

Why should we tolerate
a diet of weak poisons...?

—RACHEL CARSON

My Husband's Clover Plants: or, Why We Farm Organically

TRISH CRAPO

IT'S EARLY MARCH. My husband and I are down in the second greenhouse. The day is damp, overcast; what light there is arrives through the layers of two-year-old plastic in a shadowless, confused way. Outside, a few birds trill the same note back and forth.

The greenhouse is a mess; strings of red baling twine used to tie up last season's tomato plants dangle from the ceiling, rolls of snow fence curl on their cinder block supports, undoing the make-shift benches. Mice have obviously tunneled in and gnawed at the foam insulation along the north wall. My husband takes a rake and teases long, dead weeds from the gravel floor, stirring up grey dust. All the little details neglected in the rush of harvest and farmers' markets last fall must now be attended to. It's spring cleaning time; time to start the first trays of seeds.

This year, my husband says, the first trays will be echinacea, even though last year's plants never made it into the ground. In the rush of transplanting last spring, more tried and true market crops prevailed over this experimental newcomer. The failure of last year's echinacea crop, however, doesn't deter my husband. You only have so much time, he says. You have to make choices. You do what you can; you learn from your mistakes. You go on. Watching him work, with an unhurried ease that seems almost a physical meditation, it occurs to me that each small, mechanical task in farming is an expression of hope. Against all odds—by which I mean aphids, mice, grasshoppers and leaf-hoppers, nemotodes, fungus, heavy winds, drought, flood; not to mention the national economy—my husband grows food. Even more amazing, he does it organically, using no chemical pesticides, fungicides or fertilizers. Year after year, he produces luscious tomatoes; shiny, dark zucchini; the sweetest of sweet corns; lettuces so beautiful you could give one to your sweetheart as a bouquet (I've received several!). The bounty of our little farm continues to amaze me.

In the greenhouse, my husband and I are talking about why he does this. It's me, the writer, asking. Obviously, he's not in it for the big bucks, I say. Neither of us have ever met an organic farmer who made big bucks. (But hey, if you're out there, all power to you!) And even before the current wrangling over national organic regulations, organic standards in our state, Massachusetts, were detailed and demanding, often frustrating to keep up with year after year. You'd finally hit on a greenhouse soil mix that worked and invariably some crucial ingredient was banned from organic production the next year. Yet, our farm was one of the first in the state to be certified by NOFA/MASS (the Massachusetts chapter of the Northeast Organic Farming Association), in 1986, the first year of its certification program, and my husband has kept up his organic certification ever since.

"Why bother?" I ask, ever the devil's advocate. "I mean, it's so much work to grow organically; it's kind of expensive; you have to follow so many rules! It's a moral thing, right?" My husband keeps raking.

"It's the principle of it," I say, persisting. "It's because you believe in it."

My husband rakes. "See this?" he says, finally, touching the first fisted leaves of a clover plant with the tines of the rake. "See this clover plant right here? This clover plant reminds me of why I do it."

Every year for three years, since he put up this greenhouse, my husband tells me, the same three clover plants keep making their way back, shoving through the thick layer of stones, leaning to grow out from under an ill-placed cement block, putting up with dry heat, wet heat, the indignity of powdery mildew every fall. These tenacious plants overcome any curve ball my husband or the growing season can throw them, and my husband has begun to look forward to seeing them every year; he's actually started to plan his greenhouse set-up around them.

I stare at the floor of the greenhouse. "Okay," I say. Then, lunging into the riddle of my husband's clover plants, I draw a breath and ask him, "Is it about 'husbandry?' 'Stewardship?' Taking care of the land?

Is it about the regenerative powers of nature? About, you know, Mother Earth?"

My husband is quiet for a minute. "Sort of," he says, but he's resisting me.

ᕋ

THE FIRST YEAR we started farming, we had so little equipment and so little expertise that a friend and I had to get down in the furrow my husband was plowing and shove over the huge, heavy ribbon of sod with our shoulders. Actually, "ribbon" is the wrong word: this thing was as big as a sidewalk. Even as we accomplished the flip of our one little section, the tractor sputtered on ahead of us, carving out more and more sidewalk, maybe enough to walk to China on! My friend and I were like woodblock print people at first, workers in a Socialist Realist poster rising nobly to our task, muscling the earth over. Then, all of a sudden, what we were doing, though still obviously necessary, struck both of us as ridiculous—outdatedly Herculean—and as we struggled we got to laughing at each other, grunting around down in a big slot in the ground. My friend had an earthworm in his beard; I had a couple in my hair. It was 1981. I was twenty-three years old. I had never been so dirty or laughed so hard in my life.

ᕋ

OF COURSE, as the years went on we became more experienced as farmers, which is to say the problems we encountered became more complicated. We'd no sooner get aphids under control—no problem, use a soap spray or release ladybugs—than we'd develop some kind of puckery red leaf curl we'd never seen in any organic gardening book. We'd think we had our marketing nailed down—a season commitment from a major natural foods chain—and then California organic lettuce would come in at half our price and it turned out what we had was a verbal agreement, not a contract. One ill-timed rainy day at market in the middle of, say, sweet corn season, could wreak complete havoc with all of those careful income projections my husband spent most of January putting together.

The puzzles and rigors of organic farming required more than enthusiasm; they called for research, creative thinking, stick-to-it-iveness, and in some cases, bank loans. The purchase of a mechanical transplanter in 1990 moved us into the modern age (though admittedly, just the early end of the spectrum, like say, the 1950's) and virtually put an end to my husband's trips to the chiropractor. Dropping the plants into this ferris wheel contraption was satisfying and fun; each time the machine closed the gap in the soil around the transplant and squirted it with fish emulsion tea I was newly amazed. Look at what this machine can do! To think we had spent years dragging flats of transplants down these rows (hadn't they been longer then?) scrabbling around on our hands and knees, gouging at the dirt with trowels, praying for rain that hardly ever came.

The transplanter, and other equipment purchases we made over the years, increased our productivity and made us feel more like real farmers. We were getting somewhere with this organic farm thing; we could handle more acreage. Having the appropriate equipment gave us a more even footing in the mammoth balancing act we were trying to perform—an act which included as co-performers a quarter acre of raspberries, the same of asparagus, five to seven acres of mixed crops for sales to farmers' markets, local groceries and restaurants, and ten acres of hay, pasture and Christmas trees, as well as every organism already occupying every inch of that land. Our equipment inventory to date includes "Little John," an older high-clearance cultivating John Deere tractor, a plow, a harrow, a Rotovator, a manure spreader, a mower, a subsoiler, a cultivator, several hand seeders of various makes and vintage, a wheel hoe, a small arsenal of hoes of all shapes and sizes (we're always curious to try any variation of this most important of hand tools)—oh—and "Big John," a brand new John Deere four-wheel-drive tractor just off the assembly line and delivered to our farm one happy day less than a month ago. You should see how orderly the fields look right now—all of them plowed and rotovated, the soil crumbly and black as cake!

ֲ&

RIGHT NOW THE only animal on our farm is our older daughter's pygmy goat, Charlotte. Before we'd even found a piece of land for our farm, however, we fully intended to raise animals. An ideal farm, we thought, would be a holistic enterprise involving plants, animals and people. One of the problems we saw in conventional agriculture was that it ignored the ecosystem altogether, treating the soil as a convenient holding mechanism for plants. Fertility, in this way of thinking, was not something you maintained or created, it was something you brought in from the outside. Animals, we believed, helped close the loop. Besides, we were curious what it meant to raise animals.

We started with one pig, which we fed on slop from the restaurant where my husband worked nights. This pig was part pet, part walking cuts of pork. I often looked at the butchering diagram in *My Joy of Cooking* to remind myself of this. We named him Arnold, and he lived in a jerry-rigged pen in the backyard where we spent a fair amount of time leaning over the fence, scratching him behind the ears with a stick. Every once in a while, he'd tunnel out and have to be chased back into the pen. But, all in all, taking care of Arnold was easy. And though the trip to the slaughterhouse was sad, in the end he made a smashing Easter ham.

Gaining confidence, we bought a litter of seven pigs and a dairy cow, Celeste. At various times over the next five years we had as many as twenty pigs and a "herd" of seven cows (in our rural town, seven cows doesn't really qualify as a herd). But as bucolic as the cows looked in the pasture, our ideal farm was turning out to be less than ideal.

When we had animals, we were always haying when we should have been transplanting, or transplanting when we should have been haying. Oftentimes, my husband would end up spending entire afternoons lying around under the baler trying to figure out what was wrong with it when he should have been *either* haying or transplanting. And in the meantime, weeds kept on growing and cabbage moths kept on laying eggs in the broccoli. What we had envisioned as a well-functioning organism was, quite frankly, a mess. It turned out that, if we wanted to succeed at being organic farmers, we had to put aside our preconceived notions of what an organic farm was, and instead figure out what we and the specific piece of land we inhabited were capable of doing together.

Similarly, years ago we tried to grow carrots. Carrots looked pretty on a farmer's market stand, expanding our color scheme, and they could be timed to come in both early and late, thereby extending our growing season. In many ways, carrots made sense. Not to our soil, however. Classified by a local extension agent as "clayey loam," our soil was a heavy pudding when wet, hard-baked as cement when dry, and riddled with stones of every size from pebbles to boulders. We grew carrots, all right, but not the nice, straight, perfectly tapered ones we'd admired in the seed catalogues. We got carrots with three or more folded roots growing from one top, carrots entangled in all manner of embrace, stubbly carrots, almost square or round ones, and carrots that were plenty long but pale as a parsnip and no bigger around than a pencil. It took a lot of time to clean some of those corkscrew carrots. We fed a lot of them to our pigs. Finally, we gave up. We had *battled* the land over those carrots, and the land had won. A neighbor, another organic farmer with whom we had marketed cooperatively over the years, grew fine carrots. And we let him do it.

From time to time, now that sixteen years of composting has lightened our soil's texture, as well as our attitude towards what we might be capable of accomplishing, my husband considers growing carrots again. And he and my daughter talk about getting farm animals. Sometimes it's a pig, sometimes a couple of cows. My husband has always wanted to have a buffalo, but my daughter is dubious.

"What would you do with a buffalo?" she asks.

"What do you do with a pygmy goat?" my husband answers.

Nothing it turns out. Absolutely nothing—unless you count feeding it, petting it every day and watching it eat grass. Which, when it comes right down to it, adds up to more than you might think.

≈

AT THE FARMERS' markets in the Boston area—now the main outlets for our produce—we've developed a reputation for quality. Though some customers come to our stand specifically seeking organic food, to many others the fact that our vegetables are organic is secondary. They notice how beautiful they are first. My husband grows sixty-five varieties of tomatoes, many of them heirlooms, and his stand is always an absolute knock-out. In this, organic farming has come a long way from the days back in the seventies when imperfection was almost a sign of the authenticity of certain organic produce. This was especially true if you came across the produce in question in a food co-op or "natural" food store. No longer a novelty, organic foods are making their way into the mainstream. Statistics from the Organic Trade Association show sales of organic foods in the U.S. at 3.5 billion dollars in 1996; and though this is still a mere 5.2% of the overall food and beverage market, it represents a tripling in six years—from 1.0 billion in 1990.

The surge of interest in organic produce has several forces driving it, I think. One is an increased interest in personal health, in what we put into our bodies and the bodies of our children. This interest can be seen manifested in tougher labeling requirements for food of all kinds. More and more we want to know, as consumers, what exactly it is we are consuming. Another factor is a renewed and strengthened interest in what we used to refer to in the seventies as "ecology," but is now most often expressed as a understanding of the need to preserve "biodiversity." The interconnected nature of the planet and its various life forms is becoming more a staple of our national consciousness—I hope I am not overly-optimistic in believing this. Even if the trend extends less beyond my own geographical boundaries than I think it does, the experience of the past sixteen years tells me we are, in fact, making progress.

Every time a customer walks up to our tables at the farmers' market and stands there trying to decide what to buy, there is an opportunity to spread the word about what organic means. I often think that perhaps the most compelling reason to grow anything organically is, in fact, the simple fact that someone else is going to eat it. There's a sacred kind of trust you enter into with your customers. I have grown this in a way that won't hurt you, you seem to be saying to them when you display your "certified organic" seal. Yet, there is always at least one customer at any given market who asks, "Why would you have to grow flowers, (or Jack-o-lantern pumpkins, or decorative gourds...) organically?" You're not going to eat them, the question implies. So there's more to it than that.

≥≥

I used to ask my husband what would happen if really big farms—"agribusiness"—got into organic agriculture. This notion actually seemed somewhat unlikely in the mid-eighties, but I thought we ought to be mentally prepared for it anyway. The price structure could go all to pieces, it seemed to me, and the dedicated, pioneering growers who had been patiently producing organic food for so many years would be shoved out of the market. Green beans seemed one clear-cut example: we knew how labor-intensive it was to pick beans. It took the two of us most of an entire day to pick twelve to fourteen bushels, which was a drop in the bucket compared to what agribusiness was capable of producing. We charged ten to twelve dollars a bushel for our beans, and they were lovely—always long, perfect, young, organically grown green beans. A mechanical bean-picker, or even a contraption whereby six or eight teenagers could lie on their stomachs on a mattress and be transported down the bean rows all of them picking, could easily drop the price to $6.00–8.00. And this confused me. Steeped in the "Food for People, Not for Profit" atmosphere of the more radical food co-ops of the 1970's, I was hopelessly in conflict with myself. I suspected I was the enemy. Of course I wanted people to have inexpensive organic food; but now that I was involved in doing it, it turned out food (organic or not) was pretty expensive to produce! It took a lot of time; it was a lot of hard work; and sometimes, when a crop failed or frost came a little earlier than you'd expected, it broke your heart, not to mention your pocketbook.

My husband, though, said that if agribusiness entered organic farming to such an extent that he was driven out, he'd know for sure that he'd done what he set out to do. Organic agriculture as the norm? All over America, maybe all over the world? Sure—isn't that what we wanted? Besides, he didn't think he'd ever be completely driven out. There'd always be something he could grow, some crop that was too labor-intensive for agribusiness to bother with, too perishable or finicky, too inconvenient in some way you couldn't even think of just yet. There'd always be some little niche. And this is good—since I can't imagine my husband not growing something.

&

IT'S MID-APRIL. Down in the greenhouse both doors are open and it's 90 degrees inside. The baling twine's been untangled; draped and clipped to the greenhouse supports. Super Chilis and tomatoes, onions and flowers are up. The transplanting chores are increasing at breakneck speed. Right in the greenhouse "floor" short rows of baby lettuce and mixed greens and spinach are flourishing, providing us with delicious salads. The experiment probably won't lead to a crop of mesclun next year, though. We now know why these greens sell for eight to nine dollars a pound—it takes forever to pick them and even longer for them to amount to anything in volume! Better to pick a handful and put it right in your mouth, to pick a bagful and give it to a neighbor, than to pile up too many chores all in the same few precious weeks of spring. Under the benches, well, they're still there— my husband's clover plants—big and bushy and green. As far as I can tell, for as long as we live here, those clover plants are going to be there. My husband's hell-bent on it. That's his job.

"The pace of industrialization of agriculture has quickened. The dominant trend is a few, large, vertically integrated firms controlling the majority of food and fiber products in an increasingly global processing and distribution system. If we do not act now, we will no longer have a choice about the kind of agriculture we desire as a Nation."

A TIME TO ACT: A REPORT OF THE USDA
NATIONAL COMMISSION ON SMALL FARMS

"Small farms cannot exist in a vacuum as relics of days gone by preserved for the tourists or nostalgia for how most everyone's great grandparents lived. Small farms are a vital functioning part of a working landscape that includes Jeffersonian entrepreneurs of all kinds—locally owned grocery stores, garages, machinery dealerships and other business operating on a similar scale as the farmers they both serve and depend on."

CLARK HINSDALE, VERMONT FROM THE PUBLIC TESTIMONY
QUOTED IN A TIME TO ACT: A REPORT OF THE USDA NATIONAL
COMMISSION ON SMALL FARMS

The Structure And Character Of American Agriculture

- Nearly half of U.S. land is farmland, over one billion acres. Only 4% of landholders hold 47% of this farmland.†
- The U.S. has 300,000 fewer farms than in 1979. §
- Less than 2% of the nation's population is engaged in farming. §
- Approximately 60% of all farms are less than 180 acres in size. §
- Small farms (farms which gross under $250,000) make up 94% of U.S. farms. §
- Up until the 1950's, the economy of rural America was based primarily on agriculture. Today, agriculture is the dominant industry in only one-fourth of rural counties. §
- From 1980–1990 80% of farming-dependent counties lost population, and farm jobs declined by 111,000. §

- The 18- to 34-year-old population in farming-dependent counties declined 17% on average from 1980–1990. §
- Figures from the 1992 Census show that: 25% of U.S. farmers are 65 years of age or older; between 1982–1992 the percentage of young farmers under 25 dropped by half; the average age of the American farmer was 53 years old. §
- USDA research predicts that between 1992 and 2002, a half million farmers will retire—approximately 25% of all farmers. Only 250,000 farmers are predicted to replace them. §

Economic Status Of Small Farms In America

- Nationwide, 7% of American farms received 60% of the net cash farm income in 1992.†
- Small farms (farms which gross under $250,000) make up 94% of U.S. farms, yet receive only 41% of all farm receipts. In other words: out of 2 million farms, only 122,810 of the super-large farms receive the majority of receipts. §
- Direct marketing opportunities for small farms have increased in recent years; most notably in the form of farmers' markets. In 1994, the USDA National Farmers Market Directory listed 1,755 markets; two years later it listed 2,400. §
- The USDA Commission on Small Farms found that small family and part-time farms are at least as economically efficient as large operations, and contribute more in "public values" to our society. ("Public values" include diversity, environmental benefits, self-empowerment and community responsibility, places for families, and the development of meaningful consumer connections to food) §

Government Support For Small/Family Farms

- In 1992, 68% of U.S. government farm payments went to the wealthiest 19% of agricultural producers.†
- In 1995, the 11% of small farms with gross sales between $100,000 and $249,000 received 28% of commodity program payments. Large farms (6% of all farms) received 31% of commodity program payments. Small farms averaged payments of approximately $11,000 per farm, while large farms received

an average of $20,000 per farm. The larger the farm, the larger the payment. §

Government Support For Organic/Sustainable Agriculture

• USDA Research projects rated as "Strong Organic" by OFRF (Organic Farming Research Foundation) represent less than one-tenth of one percent of USDA's research portfolio, both numerically and fiscally.*

• According to a 1993 self-review by the USDA Agricultural Research Service, only about 1% of its research budget was for sustainable agriculture research.†

Burn down your cities and leave our farms,
and your cities will spring up again as if by magic,
but destroy our farms and the grass will grow
in the streets of every city in the country.

—WILLIAM JENNINGS BRYAN

The earth is given as common stock for man to labor and live on. . .
The small landowners are the most precious part of the state.

—THOMAS JEFFERSON

When we see the land
as a community to which we belong,
we may begin to use it
with love and respect.

—ALDO LEOPOLD

Soil Fertility and Animal Health

QUOTATIONS FROM THE WRITINGS OF PROF. WILLIAM ALBRECHT, CHAIRMAN OF THE DEPT. OF SOILS, UNIVERSITY OF MISSOURI, CI. 1958.

Since only the soil fertility, or that part of the soil
made up of the elements essential for life,
enters into the nutrition by which we are fed,
we may speak of animal health as premised
on soil fertility.

&

But animals must feed on organic substances.
They take to bulky vegetation, such as grass, hay, etc.,
and not to salts and minerals except as "an act of desperation"…
They search out better nutrition, even at the risk of their lives.

&

Many of the organic feed compounds demanded by animals
are the same as those required by plants
for their growth, reproduction and survival.

&

Nature uses no concentration salts
in building up her soils to an ecological climax.
Instead she uses the decaying organic matter
of the past dead generations
of exactly the same plant species which she is growing.

&

The microbes are the first crop we grow every spring.

&

Only by fertile soil can there be created ample supplies
of the complete proteins by which not only growth
but protection as health, and reproduction as survival
of the species are concerned.

Sustainable Food System Approaches to Improving Nutrition and Health

GERALD F. COMBS, JR.,[1] ROSS M. WELCH[2,3] AND JOHN M. DUXBURY[3]. REPRINTED FROM *AGRICULTURAL PRODUCTION AND NUTRITION: PROCEEDINGS OF AN INTERNATIONAL CONFERENCE*, BOSTON, MA, MARCH 19-21, 1998 BY PERMISSION OF THE AUTHORS.

The health and well-being of every person depend on access to sustenance provided by food systems of varying complexity. Yet, these systems have evolved with little explicit attention to the quality of their nutrient outputs or to their overall ability to support good health. Poor nutrition diminishes the quality of life for billions of people, particularly the poor in developing areas of the world. Therefore, we believe that to offer the poor a reasonable chance for healthier lives, it will be necessary to exploit the potentials of improved food systems. This will require changes in thinking about agriculture, health, and national development.

Impacts of Malnutrition in Today's World

Food- and nutrition-related problems are national development issues. Malnutrition affects nearly half the world's population: some 840 million people do not have access to enough food to meet their basic needs; an estimated 2 billion people live at risk of disease resulting from deficiencies of vitamin A, iodine, and iron, most of them women and children living in less developed countries; and more than a third of the world's children fail to reach their physical and mental potentials because of inadequate diets. Malnutrition decreases worker productivity and increases morbidity and mortality rates; by potentiating infectious disease, it accounts for as much as half of all child deaths. All these effects compromise the abilities of people to compete for their livelihoods, leading to continuing cycles of poverty among the disadvantaged (Combs et al., 1996).

Malnutrition is also a consumer and a public health issue. Even the United States, with the world's most plentiful and safe food supply and its most complex food system, has prevalent diet-related health problems (Barefield, 1996; Frazão, 1996; Kantor, 1996). Improper diet is recognized as contributing to at least five leading causes of death (heart disease, cancer, stroke, diabetes, and atherosclerosis). An estimated one-fifth of pre-menopausal American women are anemic, in part because of poorly bioavailable dietary iron. Low intake of calcium contributes to bone disease among women. Child growth retardation and deficiencies of vitamins A and C are prevalent among Hispanic and African Americans of lower socioeconomic status. Prevalences of overweight and obesity are increasing. These problems erode the quality of life and have substantial social and economic costs. Because the U.S. economy and global stability are also affected by food-related problems in other parts of the world, and because food security will be increasingly threatened by the expected addition of 2.5 billion people over the next 25 years, food, nutrition and health also are political and national security issues.

Linking Human Nutrition Needs to Food Systems

The traditional approaches to addressing human food and nutrition needs have been through programs targeted either to increasing the production of staple foods or to correcting specific nutrient deficiency diseases. These approaches have been conceived along either agricultural or medical lines with narrow foci and limited objectives. Such sectoral approaches tend to deal inadequately with truly complex issues; thus, most have not proven sustainable.

The best known agricultural approach to combating malnutrition was the "Green Revolution." That effort, implemented through the coordinated efforts of the consultative Group for International Agricultural Research and various national agricultural research organizations, developed technologies that allowed many developing nations to realize impressive gains in the production of staple grains (rice, wheat, and maize). Its results were dramatic: rice and wheat production in South Asia increased by 200% and 400%, respectively, within three decades; the daily global availability of food energy per capita rose to about 2720 kcal, some 16% above minimum needs (UNACC-SN, 1992a). But the current adequacy of global food production, serious maldistribution problems notwithstanding, should not be cause for comfort. The world population, now numbering 5.9 billion, is growing at an estimated annual rate of 1.7% and is expected to double within the next 40 years. To meet the demands of this growth, further large increases in agricultural production must occur.

Despite its successes, the Green Revolution served to reduce agricultural diversity, with unfortunate health outcomes. With favorable economic returns, farmers in the best agricultural environments rapidly adopted green revolution technologies, and the new, simpler, cereal-based cropping systems displaced more diverse, traditional ones that despite their lower calorie-protein outputs, provided foods with higher contents of essential micronutrients (vitamins and minerals), such as pulses (beans, peas, and lentils). Cereals, in comparison, provide meager amounts of vitamins and essential minerals; these are found moistly in the bran and germ, which are removed during milling, producing foods deficient in these nutrients. Displacement of nutrient-rich traditional crops has been exacerbated by the failure of plant breeders to produce high-yielding varieties of those crops. This can be seen in South Asia, where the production of pulses is now only 87% of what it was 30 years ago (UNACC-SN, 1993); UN-FAO), 1997). The production of fruits and vegetables also has not kept pace with population growth. The results are lower availabilities and higher prices for micronutrient-rich foods, factors that limit their accessibility, particularly for low-income families.

The nutritional impacts of reduced agricultural diversity are clear: the availability of food iron in South Asia dropped from 6.2 mg/kcal in 1970 to 5.7 mg/kcal in 1988, while the incidence of anemia among pre-menopausal women increased from about 57% in 1977 to over 73% in 1987 (UNNACC-SN, 1992a,b). In fact, the incidence of anemia among South Asian women is 1.6 times greater than that among sub-Saharan African women, who, despite their higher prevalence of calorie-protein insufficiency, have greater access to dietary iron (UNNACC-SN, 1992b). This phenomenon is seen on a global scale;

the prevalence of anemia among all women has risen from 30% in 1980 to over 40% today (Uvin, 1994). Although anemia can have several causes, including physiological iron losses in women and iron losses due to bleeding caused by parasitism or enteric disease, low intake of poorly available dietary iron from plant sources is a significant contributor. Indeed, the prevalence of low iron status is thought to be as much as twice that of anemia.

Therefore, while continued population growth makes it imperative to find ways to continue increasing agricultural production, focusing on staple food crop production alone is likely to increase micronutrient malnutrition. Micronutrient deficiencies can be overcome by including pulses or animal products in diets along with vegetables and fruits, but the poor often depend almost exclusively on low-cost staples; for example, polished rice provides over 85% of food energy for people in Bangladesh (Nazmul Hassan, personal communication, 1996). Solving these problems, therefore, will call for strategies that address issues of food nutrient bioavailability and balance.

Evidence is mounting that high-input, green revolution agricultural technologies may not be sustainable (Brown, 1995, 1996; Ross, 1996). To support their high yields, the green revolution varieties require irrigation and costly fertilizers, fuel, and pesticides. High yields, therefore, are not realized by subsistence farmers who cannot afford high inputs; the green revolution varieties selectively offer advantages to larger-scale farming operations that can afford them.

While agriculture has seen malnutrition as an issue of food availability, much of the health community has treated malnutrition like a disease. Accordingly, interventions have generally followed medical models, focusing on the proximate and evident causes of malnutrition in treating symptoms and therefore targeting specific nutrients. Health-based, sectoral interventions have thus had limited long-term impacts. Most have relied on food processing and pharmaceutical technologies, such as the use of food fortificants and specific nutrient supplements. While many such efforts have been successful, at least initially, in developing countries they frequently have met insurmountable economic, political, social, and logistical barriers, and their costs have made them dependent on international support.

An example of an unsustainable intervention program is Sri Lank's Thriposha (triple nutrient) program, which was designed to supply energy, protein and micro-nutrients free of charge to poor mothers and children in a pre-cooked, cereal-based food (PHNFLASH, 1995). Started in 1973, the program was administered through school systems and maternal-child clinics and became an important part of the country's public health effort. Yet it never reached its goals of providing nutrients to the truly needy, promoting local production of indigenous foods, and introducing an inexpensive, protein-rich foods and in some households was consumed preferentially by men. Some families maintained their eligibility for the supplement by keeping their children underweight. Some mothers used the supplement as a food replacer, and therefore did not increase the nutrient intakes of their children. Last year the Thriposha program was discontinued.

Clearly, better approaches are needed to meet the increasing nutritional demands of an expanding global population. We believe that a new agenda for food and agricultural development is needed, one for a "greener revolution" directed at increasing the production of nutritionally adequate food supplies in ways that protect biological, socio-economic, and political environments and thus ensure sustainability. To accomplish this, we believe that both agriculture and nutrition must be viewed in the larger context of their inherent interrelationships. Therefore, we convened a highly diverse group of experts from many disciplines, sectors and countries to develop such a new agenda. That group did so on the basis of a *Food System* concept that held human health and well-being as explicit outcomes (Combs et al., 1996).

We believe that the Food System concept can facilitate the development of food-based strategies for preventing malnutrition. The concept encompasses all activities relating to the production, acquisition and utilization of food; it holds food systems as varied, complex, multicomponent systems with multiple inputs (labor, capital, knowledge, seed stock, etc.) and multiple outcomes, including the health and well-being of people within such systems. It considers these activities within several subsystems: *production* (including land use and tenure; soil management; crop breeding, selection and management; livestock breeding and management; and harvesting); *acquisition* (including food processing, transportation, storage, packaging and marketing; household purchasing; and food use traditions, practices and distribution); and *utilization* (including food preparation, processing and cooking; household food decision-making; food preferences; and access to health care, sanitation, energy, and knowledge). The model holds the health and well-being of individuals as outcomes of these complex, nested subsystems interacting to varying degrees within biophysical, social, economic, public health and policy environments. From this perspective malnutrition is seen as a food systems failure.

Developing Food Systems Approaches to Micronutrient Malnutrition

We believe that the development of sustainable solutions to malnutrition, in both developing and industrialized countries, can best be addressed using systems approaches that conceive of objectives in multidisciplinary terms and take comprehensive views of both ends and means. While the agricultural sector historically has measured its success in terms of production, food systems approaches would expand that view to include measures of impacts on human nutritional and health status. Food systems approaches would identify the root causes of malnutrition and look broadly at food systems in the development of sustainable solutions.

To realize the potential of food systems to prevent malnutrition, it will be necessary to enunciate the values and foci that would direct such approaches. In addressing micro-nutrient malnutrition, we suggest that these values should include: increasing the physiological utilization of nutrients with prevalent deficiencies (e.g., vitamin A, iron, iodine, zinc); increasing the efficiency of resource utilization for nutrient production, reaching high-risk population groups; and being sustainable from environment, social, and economic perspectives. We also propose that food systems approaches be focused on the staple foods most important in diets of the poor: beans, cassava, rice, wheat, and maize. To this end, we see three approaches as most appropriate: increasing the production of micronutrients; reducing the losses of micronutrients; and increasing the physiological utilization of micronutrients.

Increasing micronutrient production

Wheat cultivars vary in their ability to thrive on soils with poorly available iron and zinc; this suggests that we can overcome limitations imposed by low availability of soil minerals in many parts of the world by breeding for increased efficiency of mineral uptake (Graham and Welch, 1996). Zinc-enhancement of seed, achieved experimentally by foliar or soil application of the element to wheat plants, has been found to increase the viability and vigor of next-generation seedlings (Welch, 1993). This suggests that the development of zinc- or iron- enriched genotypes many have important agronomic benefits (e.g., lower seeding rates, reduced fertilizer needs, increased disease resistance, increased water use efficiency, improved grain yield) besides enhanced micronutrient contents in the edible grain. Such linkages to economically important traits will be important if enhanced micronutrient contents are to be added to breeding strategies. For rice and wheat, which are milled, it will be necessary to determine whether breeding can improve endosperm mineral contents; this may be possible if ways can be found to control tissue-specific expression of genets for such compounds as phytoferritin and leghemoglobin. Loss of aleuronal minerals is not a concern for beans or for grains such as maize, unpolished rice, and wheat, which can be consumed without milling; the finding of a multiple aleurone layer gene in maize shows the potential to increase micronutrient contents of at least some species. Plant breeding may also be able to increase the vitamin contents of staple foods (e.g., rice with significant pro-vitamin A carotenoid content); genetic engineering methods may offer opportunities to transfer genes for such traits across species (e.g., developing rice containing beta-carotene).

Micronutrient output also can be enhanced by diversifying food systems. This can be approached through nutrition education and social marketing to affect food-related behavior and deployment of household resources; such efforts must be linked to measures to increase access to micronutrient-rich foods. Approaches necessarily will vary according to local circumstances; many will call for re-diversifying food systems through the introduction of micronutrient-rich crops into crop rotations. Approaches such as including early maturing legumes in rotations of rice or rice-wheat can increase the availability of pulses while returning to the soil the nutrients needed to reverse stagnating cereal productivity. Home gardening efforts emphasizing vegetables and fruits will continue to be important. However, to have positive impacts, they must address the constraints to food production in resource-poor areas: extremes in temperature and water availability, unavailability of planting materials, infertile soils, the need for protection from livestock, and demands on women's time.

Reducing micronutrient losses

Micronutrient losses from food systems can be reduced by finding effective means of using the iron- and zinc- containing cereal brans. Bran retention from wheat can be increased by producing higher extraction flours; the success of this approach depends on consumer acceptance of the coarser products. Promotion of unpolished rice or food uses of rice polishings will call for finding ways to stabilize the highly unsaturated lipids contained in the bran. Key to these efforts will be to optimize fuel use for such activities as cooking and parboiling. Gains in this areas, to the extent that they reduce use of brans as fuel, can increase their availability for food use or for recycling either as soil amendments or through animals as feeds.

Increasing the physiological utilization of micronutrients

Micronutrients utilization from plant foods can be increased by reducing phytates, the nondigestible (for humans and monogastric livestock) complexes of iron, zinc, phosphorus and calcium in plants. Recent evidence suggests the possibility of breeding reduced-phytate soybeans and corn kernels (USDA-ARS, 1996; Victor Raboy, personal communication, 1995). However, because phytates are storage forms of minerals in seeds and grains, there are questions about the impacts of such reductions on seed vigor and crop productivity. A better approach may be to develop sources of phytases, the enzymes that break down phytates, for us in food engineering and diet formulation. This can be done by germinating wheat, which activates the expression of endogenous phytases, before food use, or by processing grains in ways that facilitate their fermentation by phytase-containing fungi. Also, fungi that produce heat-resistant phytases have been cloned.

The enteric absorption of iron and zinc can be enhanced by ascorbic acid and promoter substances in meats. Ascorbic acid reduces ferric iron to the more absorbable ferrous form and stabilizes ferritin post-absorptively to enhance the bioavailability of both nonheme (plant) and heme (animal) forms of iron. The presence of meats in a meal enhances the absorption of both iron and zinc; there is evidence that this effect may involve the sulfur-containing amino acids methionine and cysteine (House et al., 1996, 1997). Elucidation of the "meat factor" would allow the characteristic to be incorporated in formulated foods, to be considered in planning meals, and perhaps to be enhanced in staple food crops through plant breeding or genetic engineering.

Conclusions

We believe that institutional changes are needed to promote more effective trans-disciplinary linkages between the agricultural and health sciences and to facilitate holistic views of agriculture, food, and development. Barriers created inadvertently by narrow disciplinary orientations must be lowered by developing programs that focus on problems and reward transdiciplinary collaboration. Nutrition, health, and sustainable development must be viewed as instrumental to each other, and programs must reflect that vision. Sustainable development implies the sustaining of people; it cannot be achieved without a population that is better nourished and healthier, more vigorous and productive in all ways, not just for physical labor, but also for mental creativity, social collaboration, and civic life. This view is captured in the food systems concept: people are both the means and the ends in the food systems perspective and their well-being should be the dominant motivating and evaluative criterion for any program. Therefore, we see improving nutrition through a variety of mutually compatible and reinforcing ways as essential for any development effort. This task calls for food systems approaches.

Come forth into the light of things,
Let nature be your teacher.

—Wordsworth

Man masters nature not by force
but by understanding.

—Jacob Bronowski

No occupation is so delightful to me
as the culture of the earth.

—Thomas Jefferson

Giving Life: The Health and Environmental Benefits of Organic Foods

Wendy Gordon, M.S.

Our modern lifestyle seems to put a premium on eating quickly. Food without fuss, mess and preparation time is considered ideal. But when we choose food that is heavily processed and packaged, we are trading off the nourishment of our bodies and our senses for convenience. In doing so, we also reinforce a network of supply and demand that is destroying local communities and traditional ways of life all over the world. And we support a method of agriculture that is ecologically unsound, that depletes the soil of its nutrients, wastes energy and leaves harmful chemical residues in our food.

Perhaps the greatest gift you can give yourself, your family and the planet is to make just a few simple changes in your diet. Healthy food, grown well, nourishes the soul as well as the body. It can connect us to the earth, the seasons, the people who grow our food and the places in which it was grown. It can be "transformative," according to Alice Waters, "combining the political—your place in the world of other people—with the most intensely personal—the way you use your mind and your senses, together for the gratification of your soul."

Industrialized Farming: The Health Risks of Pesticides

An industrialized system of agriculture—one reliant on monoculture, synthetic chemicals, biotechnology and long-distance shipping—currently dominates the American food system. Powerful food conglomerates now make most of the critical decisions about what foods to produce, as well as where and how they are grown, treated and handled. Indeed, four multinational food companies now control the production and marketing of over 40 percent of four basic commodities: corn, soybeans, wheat and rice[4].

Are the best interests of the consumer being met by industrialized farming? On the surface it may appear so. Despite the dismay we may feel when we see our grocery bills, food at the point of purchase in America is among the cheapest in the world. Major food companies are able to meet the public's demand for a cheap and abundant food supply by controlling all the sectors involved in food production. Their greatest profits are tied to the sale of inputs to the farmers—costly machines, fossil fuels, synthetic pesticides, herbicides and fertilizers—and to adding value through processing, packaging and advertising[4]. Companies spend huge sums on advertising and marketing ploys in order to persuade the consumer to buy overly packaged and processed foods. They also extensively save on labor and environmental regulations by moving production out of the U.S.

Fred Kirschenmann, who organically farms 3100 acres in North Dakota, argues that "the price and convenience of conventional foods doesn't cover many of the environmental, social and medical costs attributable to modern agriculture." While these hidden costs may not be turning up in our food bill, we are paying for them in other sectors of the economy[3,4]. Pesticides are a prime case in point.

Nearly one billion pounds of pesticides are applied to U.S. farms every year[8,10]. These pesticides are not essential to agriculture. Yet because of the vulnerability of uniform, single crops to diseases and pests, monocropping has made conventional farmers dependent on chemicals[1,8].

Many pesticides approved for use by the Environmental Protection Agency were registered long before extensive research linking these chemicals to cancer and other diseases had been completed. Now the EPA considers 60 percent of all herbicides, 90 percent of all fungicides and 30 percent of all insecticides carcinogenic. Of the 28 most commonly used pesticides, at least 23 are potentially carcinogenic[9,10]. Many of these chemicals also potentially cause disturbing aberrations to our reproductive systems, and to our offspring[2,10].

The National Academy of Sciences projects 20,000 cancer deaths and thousands of new cancers per year from pesticide residues in food alone[9]. The average child receives four times the average adult exposure to at least eight widely used, cancer-causing pesticides in conventionally grown food. The rapid development of important physiological systems—such as the nervous system—during infancy and early childhood make the very young more vulnerable to pesticides' harmful effect[9,10].

A National Cancer Institute study found that farmers exposed to herbicides had six times more risk than non-farmers of contracting cancer[3]. In California, reported pesticide poisonings among farm workers have risen an average of 14 percent a year since 1973 and doubled between 1975 and 1985. Farmers in the midwest were warned in 1994 to wash their workclothes in a separate machine from their families because of the high incidence of tumors and cancers amongst wives and children of farmers[1].

Groundwater, the primary drinking water source in most rural areas, is also contaminated by farming chemicals. The EPA has found at least 90 pesticides in the groundwater of 38 states[1,10].

Beginning with DDT, banned in this country since 1972 but still in use in other countries, certain synthetic chemicals used in many pesticides have been shown to be hormone disruptors in wildlife. These include the chlorinated compounds such as dioxins, PCBs (polychlorinated biphenols) and DDE (a breakdown of DDT). Hormone-disrupting chemicals disperse throughout the worldwide environment. Declining fertility and misshapen and abnormal genitalia have been found in conjunction with exposure to PCBs, dioxin and DDE in such diverse populations as Arctic polar bears, Mediterranean dolphins and alligators in a Florida lake[2].

To date, researchers have identified at least 51 synthetic chemicals— many of them ubiquitous in the environment—that disrupt the endocrine system in one way or another. While the reproductive consequences for humans have yet to be documented, developmental problems, including lower IQs have been recorded in children of women who ate fish from the Great Lakes contaminated with PCBs[2].

During the post-World War II period, which spawned the widespread use of synthetic pesticides, rates of breast cancer, prostate cancer and endometriosis have risen alarmingly. Since 1940, a woman's lifetime risk of breast cancer has more than doubled. In Denmark, the rate of testicular cancer tripled between the 1940s and the 1980s; the same researcher, Niels Skakkebaek, found that the "average human male sperm counts worldwide had dropped by almost 50 percent between 1938 and 1990"[2].

The Promise of Organic

Farming does not need to rely so heavily on petroleum-based chemicals and inflict harm on farmers, consumers and the soil. A few pioneering farmers broke free of, or resisted, chemical dependency and established successful alternatives[1]. Thousands are now growing crops organically. Most of them don't use any synthetic pesticides and fertilizers at all. Raising crops free of chemicals often makes them less susceptible to drought and other natural disasters, and the improved soil structure that results from using organic materials like manure is also more drought-resistant. If a farmer grows a greater variety of different crops, his farm as a whole is not as vulnerable to the same pests or seasonal weather events. Because organic and sustainable agriculture is based on understanding and working with nature's systems, use of expensive pesticides, fertilizers, and machinery becomes less necessary.

It has been proven that sustainable farming systems can be as productive and profitable as conventional systems. In addition, since sustainable systems operate best on a smaller scale, and require more on-site management skills, they result in more farms and more farmers. Increases in farming activity provide economic and social benefits to rural communities.

Today, total U.S. sales of organic products are skyrocketing, increasing annually at a rate that is 5 times the rate of any other food sector. Sales reached $3.5 billion in 1996, an increase of 26.3 percent over the year before, *The Natural Food Merchandiser* reported in June 1997. Organic produce sales increased by 21 percent to $402 million.

Consumer demand is driving supply. Total organic cropland doubled nationally from 1991 to 1994, from 550,267 acres to 1,127,000 acres nationwide, according to United States Department of Agriculture (USDA) estimates. So has the number of organic farmers, from 2481 in 1991 to 4060 in 1994, according to the Organic Farming Research Foundation (OFRF).

Mainstream supermarkets are rapidly entering the organic market. Mass market sales of organic products totaled $210 million in 1995, a 22 percent increase in one year. But with grocery sales in the

U.S. totaling $412.5 billion, as reported in the *Progressive Grocer*, organic sales still represent less than 1 percent of the total.

Alternative markets—natural food stores, food buying clubs, cooperatives, community supported agriculture (CSAs) and farmers' markets—provide us with the best of the organic harvest as well as a way to bring consumers and food producers closer together. Between 1994 and 1996, farmers' markets increased 20 percent, from 1755 to more than 2400, according to the "1996 Farmers' Markets Survey Report" published by the USDA's Agricultural Marketing Service. Reflecting a similarly strong growth curve, there are in operation today at least 500 active CSAs, a direct distribution system for food between a particular farm and a set of consumers, all started since the 1980s.

Healthy Farms, Foods and Families:
By Choice, Not Chance

When we choose food grown in a way that is environmentally responsible, we are taking good care of ourselves and the planet. Few of us realize—as we race through the grocery aisles "hunting and gathering" our food for the week ahead, or maybe just for the next meal—that with our food choices, we are casting a "vote" for or against sustainable food production, a system of agriculture that nourishes the earth while providing food that best nourishes the body. But, as writer/farmer Wendell Berry says, "How we eat determines, to a considerable extent, how the world is used." Conversely, how we use the world determines how well we eat.

Mothers & Others has developed a simple check list to help you in planning your family's diet and to make healthier, greener food choices for you, your family and the world. As with organic food production, which brings ecology together with whole farm planning, our *Eight Simple Steps to a New Green Diet* brings ecology together with whole nutritional planning. It's the interrelationships that count, between our bodies, our health and the health of the planet. Here's how to shop for the earth, cook for your health and bring pleasure back to your kitchen:

1 • Eat a variety of food

When you eat a wide variety of food, a broad range of nutritional requirements is likely to be met. You also draw on biological diversity. The proliferating "variety" in supermarkets does not reflect biological variety, since so many of the hundreds of available products are made from the same relatively few raw food materials-corn, wheat, rice and potatoes. People today rely on just 20 varieties of plants for 90 percent of their food. Instead, you can eat a wider variety of whole foods instead of food novelties, whose claims to diversity are based on processing techniques and artificial colors and flavors.

2 • Buy locally produced food

The average mouthful of food travels 1,200 miles from farm to factory to warehouse to supermarket to our plates. In comparison, food available from local farms is almost always fresher, tastier and closer to ripeness. In addition, buying local products supports regional growers, thereby preserving farming near where you live, and requiring less energy for transport. Since the production of a wide variety of fruits and vegetables is more economical if the farmers have outlets for their produce nearby, local marketing should be encouraged. And, because it isn't being shipped long distances, local food is less likely to have been treated with post-harvest pesticides.

3 • Buy produce in season

Out-of-season produce is extravagant because it is so amazingly energy-intensive. It costs about 435 calories to fly one 5-calorie strawberry from California to New York. Out-of-season produce is also more likely to have been imported, possibly from a country with less stringent pesticide regulations than the U.S. Eating frozen fruits and vegetables, especially from local producers, is your very best option during the winter months. Frozen foods retain much of their nutritional content, in addition to cutting energy costs.

4 • Buy organically produced food

Organically grown means that the food has been grown in a practical, ecological partnership with nature. Organic food is minimally processed to maintain its integrity, without artificial ingredients, preservatives or irradiation. Organic certification is the public's guarantee that the product has been grown and handled according to strict procedures without synthetic chemical inputs.

5 • Eat fresh, whole foods with adequate starch and fiber.

Whole foods-including fruits, vegetables, grains, legumes (beans), nuts and seeds-are the healthiest foods we can eat. The National Cancer Institute recommends we each "strive for five" servings of fresh fruits and vegetables a day, since the complex carbohydrates and fiber they contain play a major beneficial role in protecting against cancer, heart disease and common digestive ailments.

6 • Eat fewer and smaller portions of animal products

Modern meat production involves intensive use of grain, water, energy and grazing areas. It takes about 390 gallons of water to produce a pound of beef. Almost half of the energy used in American agriculture goes into livestock production. Cattle and other livestock consume more than 70 percent of the grain produced in the U.S. and about a third of the world's total grain harvest. Animal agriculture also produces surprisingly large amounts of air and water pollution. Pork is the most resource intensive, followed by beef, then poultry. Eggs and dairy products are much less resource-intensive. Animal products, especially beef, are also a major source of fat in the U.S. diet. Reducing meat consumption and eating lower on the food chain protects us against heart disease, cancer and diabetes.

7 • Choose minimally processed and packaged foods

After it leaves the farm, food is subjected to a variety of processes (including packaging), most of which use fossil energy while removing naturally-occurring nutrients. A typical highly processed (and highly advertised) "food product" may contain on average only 7% real food. Processing provides no value to the biological variety of the diet when the refined food fraction is converted into hundreds of products high in fat, salt or sugar.

8 • Prepare your own meals at home

Cooking from scratch can involve a little more labor and a little more time, but you can be sure you'll save money and resources, because you're not paying someone else to prepare your food, to add nutrients removed in processing, to put it in a box or can, to ship it across the country, and to advertise it in slick TV commercials. You will also provide your family with healthier, more nutritious food since you are starting with fresh ingredients. And, cooking from scratch can be its own reward, providing a truly creative outlet which brings you pleasure and joy, rejuvenates the family meal, and nourishes our bodies and our souls.

The Road Ahead

Our food choices provide the nourishment and satisfaction that we want and need today, but also have an impact on how our food will be grown and processed tomorrow. Mothers & Others was motivated to create the *Eight Simple Steps to a New Green Diet* as a way by which concerned consumers could reform the industrial food system with their purchases. We consumers have power in our purchases, the power to change the system by which our food is grown. As organic farmers are demonstrating, synthetic pesticides are not necessary in food production. Great tasting food can be grown in abundance without them. It's a win-win proposition for us, the consumers, when we choose organic foods. We get great quality food with no toxic residues and are supporting a method of food production that does not harm the environment, the farmers working in the fields, or the consumers. So, give yourself a treat today; join in discovering the pleasures of organic foods.

Why Should I Buy Organic Products?

EXCERPTED FROM FRAN MCMANUS, EDITOR, *EATING FRESH FROM THE ORGANIC GARDEN STATE*. (PENNINGTON, NJ: NORTHEAST ORGANIC FARMING ASSOCIATION—N.J., 1998.

1. To protect local farms. Organic farms are typically small family farms that grow a variety of fruits, vegetables, grains, and animal products for local markets. Their existence plays an important regional economic and environmental role; a thriving community of local organic farms helps ensure the continued viability of small farms, makes productive use of open lands, and maintains diversity of land use in our state.

2. To preserve and enhance the local environment. Organic farmers work to build healthy soil that is full of living organisms and free of toxic chemicals. Synthetic pesticides and fertilizers have been identified as major sources of nonpoint pollution of streams and aquifers. Organic farmers use cultivation and crop rotation to eliminate weeds and apply natural materials to fertilize the soil, which helps keep unwanted chemicals out of local water systems. Many of the techniques used by organic farmers to enhance their soil also help to prevent erosion and runoff, thereby reducing the problems of sediment loading and nitrogen contamination in local water ways.

Organic farmers conserve natural resources in other ways. By using human energy and natural fertilizers, they reduce their reliance on fossil fuels, and by composting, they turn plant and animal waste into fertilizer for next year's crops. The humus in their soil retains moisture, thereby reducing the need for irrigation.

3. To reduce chemical pesticides in your community. Many of the pesticides now used on food crops—and approved by the U.S. EPA—are classified as probable human carcinogens. Studies of human and animal exposure have linked many pesticides to a variety of health problems, including some forms of cancer, impaired functioning of the immune system, neurological problems, and disruption of the hormones that regulate the body's sexual development. Because organic certification precludes the use of synthetic and persistent pesticides, organic farmers reduce the risk of exposure to chemical pesticides for their workers and the communities.

4. To maintain diversity in our food crops. Genetic diversity is how nature—and the organic farmer—protect against massive crop loss by disease or infestation. Conventional farms typically plant vast acreage with genetically identical seed varieties. The lack of genetic diversity means less choice for the consumer and causes our primary food sources to be more vulnerable to destruction by disease and pests. Organic growers grow a variety of crops that are rotated on a regular basis. They grow antique and heirloom varieties that are chosen for their flavor, genetic diversity and suitability to our climate.

5. To preserve the gene pool. In an attempt to "improve" foods, scientists are now swapping genetic material from bacteria, animals and plants. On supermarket shelves are a variety of products that have been produced with this new technology—most without any labeling that identifies them as genetically engineered. Organic farmers certification guidelines currently prohibit the use of genetically engineered products. The label is your guarantee that neither the product nor an ingredient is bioengineered.

The immune system of every unborn child in the world
will soon be adversely and irrevocably affected
by the persistent toxins in our food, air, and water.

—PAUL HAWKEN

As cruel a weapon as the cave man's club,
the chemical barrage has been hurled
against the fabric of life.

—RACHEL CARSON

Man has lost the capacity to foresee and forestall.
He will end by destroying the earth.

—ALBERT SCHWEITZER

A nation that destroys the soil destroys itself.

—FRANKLIN D. ROOSEVELT

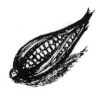

Chemicals, Plants and Man

PETER TOMPKINS AND CHRISTOPHER BIRD

In the early nineteeth century an American of English descent named Nichols cleared hundreds of acres of rich virgin land in South Carolina, on which he grew crops of cotton, tobacco, and corn so abundant that with the revenue he built a big house and educated a large family. Not once in his liftime did he add anything to the soil. When it became depleted and his crops dwindled, he cleared more land and continued his exploitation. When there was no more land to be cleared the family fortunes declined.

Nichols' son, grown to manhood, looked at the poverty stricken acreage, took Horace Greeley's advice and moved west to Tennessee where he cleared two thousand acres of virgin land; like his father he planted cotton, corn, and tobacco. When his own son was grown to manhood, the land was once more so depleted from having living things taken from it and none returned that he moved on to Horse Creek in Marengo Country, Alabama, there to purchase another two thousand acres of fertile soil and raise a family of twelve children on the proceeds; the town became Nicholsville; Nichols became the owner of a sawmill, a general store, and a gristmill. This man's son also grew up to see devastation where his father had grown rich. He decided to move further west and settled in Parkdale, Arkansas where he bought one thousand acres of good land on the bayou.

Four moves in four generations. Multiplied by thousands, this is the story of how Americans raised food on a continent which was there for the taking. The great-grandson of the original Nichols, together with thousands of other farmers, inaugurated a new era. After World War I he began by farming his new acreage, instead of just mining it, adopting the new government recommended artificial fertilizers. For a time his cotton crops prospered but soon he noticed that his pest population was much worse than it had been. When the bottom fell out of the cotton market his son Joe decided that medicine, not farming, was to be his career.

At the age of thirty-seven Joe Nichols was a full-fledged physician and surgeon in Atlanta, Texas, when he suffered a massive heart attack which nearly killed him. He was so frightened that for weeks he gave up his practice to consider his situation. All he had been taught in medical school, plus the opinions of his colleagues, suggested his prognosis was extremely doubtful. There was no answer for his affliction beyond nitroglycerin pills, which alleviated his chest pains but caused equally painful headaches. With nothing better to do than to leaf through the ads of a farming magazine, Nichols casually came across the line "People who eat natural food grown in fertile soil don't get heart disease."

"Pure quackery! Quackery of the worst sort," said Nichols of the magazine which was Organic Gardening and Farming, edited by J.I. Rodale. "He isn't even a doctor!"

Nichols remembered that for lunch on the day of his massive heart attack he had consumed ham, barbecue meat, beans, white bread, and pie, which he considered a healthy meal. As a doctor he had advised hundreds of patients on diet. But a line in the magazine nagged him: What was natural food? What was fertile soil?

At the local library the librarians were helpful in bringing Nichols books on nutrition. He also scoured the medical literature, but could find no answer to what constituted natural food.

"I had an A.B. and an M.D. degree," says Nichols, "was fairly intelligent, had read a lot, owned a farm, but I didn't know what was natural food. Like many another American who hadn't really investigated the subject, I thought natural food meant wheat germ and black molasses, and that all natural-food addicts were faddists, quacks, and nuts. I thought you made land fertile by dumping commercial fertilizer on it."

Now, more than thirty years later, Joe Nichols' thousand-acre farm near Atlanta, Texas, is one of the showplaces of the state; he has never again been afflicted with a heart attack. He ascribes both successes to the advice which he took from Sir Albert Howard's book *Agricultural Testament* and Sir Robert McCarrison's *Nutritional and Natural Health*. On his farm, not another ounce of chemical fertilizer went into the land, nothing but natural compost.

Nichols realized that all his life he had been eating "junk food," food produced from poisoned land, food that had led straight to a massive heart attack. A third book, *Nutrition and the Soil* by Sir Lionel J. Picton, convinced him that the answer to metabolic disease, whether it was heart trouble, cancer, or diabetes was indeed natural, poison-free food grown on fertile soil.

The food we eat is digested and absorbed from the intestine into the bloodstream. Essential nutrients are carried to the individual cells all over the body, where repair work is done by metabolism, the process by which stable nonliving matter is built up into complex and unstable living material, or protoplasm. The cell has an amazing capacity to repair itself provided it gets proper ingredients through proper nutrition; otherwise it becomes stunted or goes out of control. The cell or basic unit of life where metabolism occurs, needs essential amino acids, natural vitamins, organic minerals, essential fatty acids, unrefined carbohydrates, and several more as yet unknown, but presumable natural, factors.

Organic minerals, like vitamins, are found in balanced proportions in natural food. The vitamins themselves are not nutrients, but substances without which the body cannot make use of nutrients. They are parts of an extremely complex, intricately interrelated whole.

In "balance" means that all the nutrients used by the tissues must be available to the cell simultaneously. Furthermore the vitamins essential to proper nutrition and good health must be natural. There is a great difference between natural and synthetic vitamins, not a chemical but a biological difference. There is something missing in the artificial that is of biological or life-enhancing value. Not yet widely accepted, this fact has been unequivocally established by the work of Dr. Ehrenfried Pfeiffer, a biochemist and follower of the great natural scientist and clairvoyant Rudolf Steiner. Dr. Nichols thinks the Pfeiffer techniques can reveal exactly why natural foods or those containing natural vitamins and minerals and enzymes—another chemical com-

pound, of vegetable or animal origin, which causes chemical transformation—are superior to those grown and preserved with chemicals.

When Pfeiffer came to the United States at the outbreak of World
War II, and settled at Three-Fold Farm in Spring Valley, New York, he
worked out Steiner's "Biodynamic" system for making composts and
for treating the land, and set up a laboratory to investigate living things
without breaking them into chemical constituents.

Before his arrival in the United States Pfeiffer had developed in his
native Switzerland a "sensitivity crystallization method" to test finer
dynamic forces and qualities in plants, animals, and humans than
had thus far been detectable in laboratories. Dr. Steiner, who had given
a series of esoteric lectures at the Silesian estate of Count Keyserling
in the 1920's for agronomists concerned about the fall in productivity
of their crops, had asked Pfeiffer to find a reagent which would reveal what Steiner called "etheric formative forces" in living matter.
After months of tests with Glauber's salt, or sodium sulfate, and many
other chemicals, Pfeiffer discovered that if a solution of copper chlo-
ride to which extracts of living matter had been added was allowed
to evaporate slowly over fourteen to seventeen hours it would produce a crystallization pattern determined not only by the nature but
by the quality of the plant from which the extract was taken. According to Pfeiffer, the same *formative forces* inherent in the plant and acting to bring about its form and shape would combine with living
growth forces to form the pattern of crystal arrangement.

Dr. Erica Sabarth, current director of the Pfeiffer established laboratory in Spring Valley, showed the authors rows of beautiful crystal-
lizations, looking like exotic undersea corals. She pointed out how a
strong, vigorous plant produces a beautiful, harmonious, and clearly
formed crystal arrangement radiating through to the outer edge. The
same crystallization made from a weak or sick plant results in an
uneven picture showing thickening or incrustation.

Pfeiffer's method, says Sabarth, can be applied to determine the
inherent quality of all sorts of living organisms. When a forester sent
Pfeiffer two seeds taken from different pine trees, and asked if he
could detect any difference in the trees themselves, Pfeiffer submitted the seeds to his crystallization tests and found that, whereas one
crystal picture was an example of harmonious perfection, the other
was distorted and ugly. He wrote to the forester that one of the trees

should be a fine specimen, the other must have a serious defect. By return mail the forester sent Pfeiffer enlarged photographs of two grown trees: the trunk of one was mast straight; the other was so crooked it was useless for lumber.

At Spring Valley Pfeiffer developed an even simpler and less time-consuming method to demonstrate how life veritably pulsates from living soils, plants, and foods, but not from inorganic minerals, chemicals, and synthetic vitamins, which are dead. Requiring none of the complex equipment of the standard chemical laboratory, it uses circular filter paper discs fifteen centimeters in diameter, provided with a small hole in the center for insertion of a wick. The discs are laid in open petri dishes in which stand small crucibles containing a 0.05 silver-nitrate solution. This solution climbs up through the wick and spreads over the discs until it has expanded about four centimeters from the center.

From the brilliant-colored concentric patterns Pfeiffer has been able to disclose new secrets of life. Testing natural vitamin C taken from such products as rose hips, he established that the pattern of vitality was far stronger than from artificial vitamin C, or ascorbic acid. Rudolf Hsuschka, a follower of Rudolf Steiner, suggest that vitamins are not chemical compounds that can be synthetically produced but "primary cosmic formative forces."

Before his death, Pfeiffer pointed out in his own booklet Chromatography Applied to quality Testing that Goethe had stated a truth more than 150 years ago which is of the utmost importance with regard to the recognition of natural biological quality: The whole is more than the sum of its parts. "This means," wrote Pfeiffer, "that a natural organism or entity contains factors which cannot be recognised or demonstrated if one takes the original organism apart and determines its component parts by way of analysis. One can, for instance, take a seed, analyse it for protein, carbohydrates, fats, minerals, moisture and vitamins, but all this will not tell its genetic background or its biological value."

In an article, "Plant Relationships as Made Visible for Chromatography," published in the winter, 1968, issue of Biodynamics, a periodical to further soil conservation and increase fertility in order to improve nutrition and health, Sabargh stressed that the chromatographic technique "especially reveals the quality, even the living force of the organism." She added that she plans to explore the possibilities of the method not only as it applies to seeds and fruits but with regard to the roots of plants and all the other plant parts.

In modern processed foods the vitamins, trace elements, and enzymes are arbitrarily removed, mostly so as to render the food more durable. As Nichols puts it: "They remove the life, in effect, killing it, so that it will not live and die later."

੩੩

The end result of chemical farming, says Nichols, is always disease; first to the land, then to the plant, then to the animal, then to man. "Everywhere in the world where chemical farming is practiced the people are sick. The only ones to benefit are the companies that produce the chemicals."

੩੩

When Nichols realized what was happening to the country as a result of both chemical fertilization and chemical pesticides he took two steps. He went organic on his farm, and he sought other doctors and scientists who had made the same discoveries. Together they organized Natural Food Associates, of which Nichols became the first president. Their object was to start correcting the situation with a nationwide campaign to get the facts before the people, on the grounds that only an aroused public opinion could save America from poor food grown on poor soil. Nichols says he was determined to tell everyone just how to get natural food: "No matter how old you are, which sex you are, what color you are, where you live—north, south, east, or west, on an isolated farm or in a big city apartment."

੩੩

There is still hope if we get back on the track, says Nichols, if we begin to cleanse the poisons from every link of the food chain, so as to restore the country to proper nutrition and avoid the long decline that blighted North Africa and the Near East. To do so, and save the nation from metabolic disaster, says Nichols, we must change from an economy of exploitation to one of conservation. In the long run the country must give up chemical fertilizers and gradually revive the soil organically.

੩੩

We live from about eight inches of topsoil, containing earthworms, bacteria, fungi, and other microscopic forms of life, that provides us with vegetation, trees, insects, and animals. The only inexhaustible wealth is a fertile soil. Topsoil is the greatest natural resource of any nation; civilizations of the past have been destroyed when their fertile soils were lost.

&

Nichols... says that if we continue to exploit and teach exploitation of the soil here and abroad, the result will inevitably be war, just as it was when Japan went into Manchuria looking for protein from the soybean. Peace in this, says Nichols, depends on conservation of natural resources, not their exploitation.

Humankind has not woven the web of life.
We are but one strand within it.
Anything we do to the web
we do to ourselves,
all things are bound together,
all things connect.

—Chief Seattle

The insufferable arrogance of human beings
to think that nature was made solely for their benefit,
as if it was conceived that the sun had been set afire
merely to ripen man's apples and head their cabbages.

—Cyrano de Bergerac

A good farmer is nothing more or less
than a handy man with a good sense
of humus.

—E.B. White

Beyond the Romance: Human and Ecological Values of Organic Farming

BRITT BAILEY & MARC LAPPÉ, PH.D.

For one of us, Britt Bailey, organic farming conjures up days I spent on my grandmother's West Virginia farm as a child. I worked in her large organic garden down the hill from the road which led to the coal mine. She would sit down with me in the soft, composted dirt and teach me how to pull the carrots so that I would not break off the heads. She would then take me to the chicken co-op where she would teach me how to be as gentle as possible in reaching in to extract the precious eggs. They would become breakfast for the next morning. Afterwards, she would fold in the chicken droppings as a soil amendment to her vegetable patch. At dinner, I would proudly eat the salad we picked together. What a joy to be so close to the Earth! Only now do I realize how rich and diverse the living things in that garden were.

This halcyon vision is often the only image people conjure up when asked to picture organic farming. But farming organically connotes something more than an aesthetically pleasing way of tilling and harvesting. It is a way of life, one that allows crops to be produced without microecological destruction, a system that returns as much as it extracts. As such, organic agriculture stands in stark contrast to the burgeoning business of larger-scale, corporate-run farms. On such farms, supplying food typically becomes a monolithic operation dependent on the mass use of chemicals, fertilizers, and processing operations. The virtues of organic farming—its sustainability, minimal impact, and chemically clean produce—are lost in this intensified form of farming, with its dependency on chemical based fertilizers and pesticides.

Overview

When chemicals began being used in farming on a large scale in the 1940's, they were regarded as miracles. Chemicals like nitrogen-supplying *urea* and insect-suppressing *DDT* allowed the farmer to manage more land and plant more seed, and expand his acreage without having to spend more hours on the tractor. With more acreage came the need for more chemicals. Pests that once died after exposure to a particular pesticide soon become resistant leading to more potent and lethal chemicals. On the scale of the microecosystem, the pattern created was one of a tortuous cycle of life and death. Chemical death to insects and weeds; emergence of resistance in pests; more acreage being farmed; more chemical dependency; more microorganisms exposed to chemicals; more resistance emerging, stronger chemicals, and so on.

Take heavy nitrate use as a model. Such fertilizers cause abrupt shifts in invertebrate populations and cause overgrowth in of the draining waterways. For example, in North Carolina's large estuaries, where slow moving salt water is captured behind the islands of the Outer Banks, millions of fish have been found dead. The culprit is an organism known as *pfiesteria* which secretes a toxin that erodes fish epithelia and slowly paralyzes their muscles and suffocates them. *Pfiesteria* appears to take on their deadly toxin-secreting form when exposed to high levels of nitrogen and phosphorous—by-products of intensive agriculture, human sewage, and animal farming.[1]

Eventually, chemicals once confined to a limited area become pervasive. Formerly used pesticides like DDT and DDE have become ubiquitous and new ones, like heptachlor and chlordane have poisoned dairy cows and people from Hawaii to New York State.[2] Such chemicals often become part of ecosystems and find their way into our foods through distant migration. Because of agribusiness' escalating dependence on these and newer, ecologically limiting chemicals, sustainable growth may become impossible. To recapture this simple principle of intergenerational responsibility, we advocate a return to organic methods of agriculture on a widespread basis.

Some argue the sheer scale of operating conventional large farms requires that pesticides be used as a form of control. But such use exacts a high toll on the environment. Repeated chemical applications leave residues and an often depleted soil horizon. Herbicides like atrazine and simazine, and chemical fertilizers with high nitrate concentrations leach into aquifers, contaminating shallow and deep wells alike. The Environmental Protection Agency estimates 40% of the 70,000 small water systems (serving <10,000 population) are contaminated by one or more of these and related chemicals. According to a recent independent survey, pesticide residues routinely contaminate 77% of bulk-produced food crops, compared to lesser concentrations on 25% of organic produce.[3] Large-scale farms (>1,000 acres) also threaten the viable relationship of living organisms to their environment. By its nature, chemical-based farming suppresses certain organisms while allowing others to flourish. This newly imposed selection pressure disrupts traditional relationships.

Distancing Ourselves from the Land

By relying on chemicals, we are also taken further away from the source of our food. No longer are families working on farms that supply food to contiguous communities. Now, for the most part, large farms operate with massive machinery and minimal labor, and supply food to large food processing plants which then distribute their finished products nationally, and sometimes globally. As revealed by the recent epidemics of salmonella and E. coli 0157:H7, the net effect of intensification of production is to put many more people at risk of disease. Such production may also reduce nutritional value of the ultimate product and put in harms way those who gather, process, and distribute the food.

We believe large agribusinesses distance the consumer from nature. In many communities, inner city children do not know where their strawberries come from or that they have been doused with dozens of pesticides, nor that their bananas are raised abroad with potentially sterilizing chemicals and artificially preserved by potent fungicides.[1] Some strawberries have so much pesticide residue that they have been deemed by the National Academy of Science as generally unsafe for children to eat.[2] Methyl bromide, a dangerous fumigant, is also used widely on strawberry fields throughout the United

States.[3] It is an acutely toxic gas whose sole purpose is to sterilize the soil.[4] Such pesticides used not only have harmed the laborers that work during the planting and harvesting periods, but place thousands of children at risk in nearby schools. Bananas have been grown with the aid of soil sterilizing chemicals like dibromochloropropane (DBCP), and in countries like Costa Rica and Israel, the fruit may contain residues rendering them unfit for consumption. In these countries, hundreds of banana workers have filed suit maintaining they have been reproductively damaged or sterilized.

Sustainability

Organic farms utilizing living organisms (bacteria, natural fertilizers and bacterially-derived pesticides) to sustain and cycle nutrients through the ecosystem present many fewer risks and carry clear benefits. The diversity and complexity of organism interaction inherent in well-run organic farms keeps the soil horizons and micro-environment surprisingly well-balanced and healthy by maintaining microbial diversity, trace element, and nutrient mix.[5] The perception of microbial and floral diversity in organic soils reinforces the conviction of some noted researchers who believe organic farming provides a viable model for assuring long-range, sustainable agriculture.[6] Whereas typical agribusiness farms destroy bacterial species and deplete soil micronutrients, organic farming creates a system of production that replenishes soil microorganisms and nutrient quality. In a word, organic farming is sustainable.

In the context of farming, sustainability can be defined as the ability to maintain an ongoing relationship between yields and growth. Sustainability connotes a dynamic system that provides sufficient resources over several generations. In an ideal self-sustaining system, organic farming practices can create a farming system that flourishes without disrupting the complexity and functioning of the ecosystem over decades. Such a system is in marked contrast to conventional farming.

Chemical Selection

The intensive chemical reliance typical in most conventional agribusinesses extracts a heavy price on the environment. Synthetically manufactured chemicals used for agriculture not only destroy their intended target weeds and pests but disturb non-target organism habitats above and below the soil where they are sprayed. For instance, when the widely used herbicide glyphosate is used, it depletes the number of *Penicillium funiculosum*.[7] Much like the action of antibiotics, such applications may favor other microorganisms as susceptible species are diminished. In the instance of glyphosate, the total count of fungi, like *Acromonium strictum* and *Aspergillus fumigatus* may increase at the expense of more desirable species.

Many other species of fungi and bacteria are susceptible to pesticide toxicity. Such organisms comprise a rich and vital part of normal soil. According to E.O. Wilson, a few grams of soil, enough to be held between the thumb and forefinger, contain 10 billion bacteria, many of which have not been named or studied.[8] Such bacteria and surrounding nutrients play a large role in ecosystem health by chelating and methlylating heavy metals; detoxifying organic chemicals; dechlorinating halogenated polycyclic aromatic hydrocarbons; and rendering petrochemicals and other contaminants water soluble.

The basic elements of farming are thus intimately linked to sustaining microbial and elemental richness of the soil. Sufficient levels of nitrogen, potassium, and phosphorous, combined with trace elements are essential for plant growth. The crop rotation done on organic farms re-energizes the soil by replenishing these elements.

A Message?

These observations suggest we may do well to incorporate organic methods to conserve resources for future generations. Sustainable development is possible if smaller cells of activity are encouraged and farming co-operatives make decisions that provide renewable soil practices and no-till agriculture. Organic farming provides an ideal means of attaining these goals by regenerating depleted soils and microorganisms without the often catastrophic disturbance of the microenvironment caused by chemical treatments.

Organic farming is predicated on a philosophy of nature not amenable to large disturbances. Those who support the organic food movement stand by a natural ethos that believes that what is natural is best. But this philosophy is more than just an intellectual belief. It is most consistent with sustainable, reproducible, and regenerative agricultural practices. Organic farming returns to the land what it re-moves.

Too often the image of organic farming is that of hand laborers who eke from the soil minimal yields. In practice, organic farming methods can be done on mass scale—with record yields. Recent surveys provide evidence that organic farming operations can provide the yields touted by conventional agriculture. The highest per acre yields of wheat, corn, and sorghum yet achieved were from organic operations. We also believe in organic farming practices because they are safer from a toxicological viewpoint. Organic farming advocates are supporting what may be the only viable tradition to take farming into the 21st century: a method of extracting food from the soil that never depletes but always restores. When done rigorously, organic farming is a way of life that is both self-sufficient and benevolent to the land because it is harmonious with eons of plant and microbial evolution.

There is life in the ground;
it goes into the seeds;
and it also, when it is stirred up,
goes into the man who stirs it.

—CHARLES DUDLEY WARNER

Leave barbarians and beasts behind;
follow nature and return to nature.

—BASHO

The first law of ecology
is that everything is related.
to everything else.

—BARRY COMMONER

The Tradition of Organic Food

Marc Schwartz

My entrance to organic food was through the "side door." It was to be a doorway that led me on a life-long series of adventures and a doorway from which I began to see my life purpose unfold. In this chapter I would like to take you on a personal history tour of my life experiences with the organic foods industry. I will also discuss the long-term future of the organic food movement and offer some suggestions about what you can do to learn more about it. But before I begin, it might be helpful to extend the formal definition of organic agriculture given on page xii, with its broad view of the ecology and the issue of sustainability, by reviewing some specific aspects of organic food.

Organic food is food which has been grown, *processed, and handled* with no synthetic chemical application or utilization. This means that there is no contact with synthetic growth amendments, fertilizers, herbicides, pesticides, fumigants or additives from the moment the seed is planted *until the product is finally consumed.* In addition, the term means that no synthetic chemicals have been applied to the soil at least 36 months before the seed was planted. Many would have us believe that it is not possible to grow *and process* food in this way. But keep in mind that until the development of many of the synthetic biological warfare components during World War II and after, virtually all farms were organic farms. Organic farming was the convention for thousands of years, while today's "conventional farming " techniques have only been practiced for the last 50 years or so.

My belief in the feasibility of organic agriculture developed slowly. I would like to take you through time now on my journey to what might be called organic food consciousness. In the late 60s, I was an adolescent group worker dealing with inner city kids in Pittsburgh,

PA. My interest in food was unusual for that time only in the fact that I had been a vegetarian for about six years and occasionally baked my own bread. My parents had been upscale carnivores and we had consumed sirloin steak almost every day as I was growing up. I rebelled and gave up all meat at 17. My knowledge of food was pretty basic at this point. I even bought a cabbage once at 16 when my mother sent me to buy lettuce.

While at the child guidance center where I did my group work, I began to study the work of a researcher named Schacter concerning the effects of B vitamins on human behavior. Most of this work involved dosing schizophrenics with massive injections of B vitamins. This appeared to effect an improvement in behavior, as well as a lessening of schizophrenic episodes. I became curious about B vitamins and did some basic research of my own. I discovered that a large group of B vitamins was present in unrefined grains and grain products. I began to bake my own bread regularly from whole grain flours that I ground fresh daily using an ancient Japanese sourdough method. At that time there were no real whole wheat breads available in the supermarkets. I began to seriously consider the effect of the lack of B vitamins in the American diet and what the long-term implications of this lack could be.

At this time, one of my co-workers at the guidance center recommended that I try shopping at a small natural food co-op, The Oakland Food Co-op, not only to save money, but also to provide a link to whole grain products. I began to volunteer at the co-op and, eventually, I began to sell the bread that I now baked daily for several friends and myself. My career at the guidance center had reached a turning point; I had philosophical disagreements with the administration about the use of Ritalin to alter behavior, and finally, I quit my counseling job and decided to become serious about baking and selling whole-grain bread.

I began to feel that I could help more people by adding B vitamins to their diets than I ever would through group work. Hand grinding flour and using the slow sourdough method to produce bread was very difficult and time consuming, but it was satisfying and, by combining my bread sales income and the food discounts that I achieved through volunteering at the co-op, I was surviving. The wheat that I was using for my breads was organically grown wheat from either Arrowhead Mills or the Overbo brothers' farm in South Dakota. I did not yet understand what the word *organic* meant, but it had a nice ring to it. By this time, I had added granola to my repertoire of baked goods that I sold. One of my co-workers at the co-op had been baking granola at night, and I got ideas from him and from my experience with a granola that I had seen in a co-op in Berkley. The co-worker later moved to New York, baked in other peoples bakeries in off hours, and started the Good Shepherd Cereal Co, which he later sold. His was one of the early organic financial success stories.

In the fall of 1967 we moved the Pittsburgh Co-op from a crowded basement location to a bigger space upstairs. We certainly were not prepared for the growth spurt we experienced as a result of our move. Oddly enough, it was at this time that, succumbing to what was then a rampant desire by the counter-culture to withdraw to the country, the paid staff decided to leave en masse for West Virginia to form a craft co-operative. Overnight, I became the only remaining worker. I went on payroll and within 3 months, I had hired six more full-time employees. We grew exponentially every month. A great deal of this growth was driven by our commitment to organic foods. By now, I had a good working knowledge of what the chemicals used on soil, in food production, and in processing do to human bodies and to the environment. Our client base ranged from the ethnic neighborhood families that shopped at our store for the abundance of fresh produce that we offered, to philosophically motivated students who enjoyed our five different types of organic brown rice, to the health conscious yuppies. All in all, we were a vast success.

In early 1968 I had also begun to more intently study the science of milling. While looking for a supplier for buckwheat flour for the co-op, I happened upon a somewhat eccentric miller who had been practicing and refining the art of stone milling for over 45 years. I unofficially apprenticed myself to him on weekends. I also studied milling at Walnut Acres, Paul Keene's whole foods community project, whose mail order catalog continues to reach out to customers all over the country. Taking what I had learned, I set up a small milling system in the basement of the co-op so we could grind our own fresh, whole grain flours.

The late 60s were a time of much moving about among members of the counter culture. People were forever jumping in old VW buses and heading to San Francisco or to some remote rural retreat. Accordingly, I left the food co-op in the Spring of 1969 to help set up and run a distribution business in Bel Air, MD which became known as Laurelbrook Foods. My employer (Rod Coates) and his wife had been cured of high blood pressure and several other chronic ailments through natural methods introduced to them by their daughter (Dora Hawken) which had motivated them to start the business. I ran the mill, did stocking in the nighttime, and drove a delivery van into Pittsburgh, Washington D.C., and Baltimore in the daytime.

After about two months, I got the call to return to Pittsburgh to help rebuild our food co-op. It had mysteriously burned to the ground and basically we were forced to start all over again. Several of the members and staff and myself got together, rented another storefront around the corner, and began canvassing for memberships. It took us three months to rehab the entire interior and get things going financially. Pittsburgh had a co-op again—this time called Semple Street Natural Foods Co-op.

One of the important developments at this time was the formation of the Organic Growers and Buyers Association. Bob Rodale of the Rodale Institute's Organic Farm and Garden Magazine started this association to educate farmers and consumers about organic food issues. There were branches of this organization all over the country. I was part of the Pittsburgh group. We had about 15 members in our chapter ranging from an organic sheep rancher to organic herb farmers. Today, there remain at least two of these organizations. The Minnesota group, of which I am currently the Chair of the Board, has become a well-known organic certification organization with clients all over the world.

I stayed at Semple Street Co-op for about 2 more years until one of my milling mentors called me and pointed out an ad in the Millers News: there was an opening for a millwright at a mill in Minnesota. I had been through Minnesota several times and it had impressed me as one of the prime grain growing areas of North America, but also as being very flat and unappealing. However, I was keenly interested in this project because it involved a water turbine powered mill. I had always been interested in alternative and sustainable sources of power, as well as in food production. Even now, I live in a solar-powered, earth-sheltered house and still raise a large portion of my own food each year. So the water-powered mill piqued my interest. It was owned by a co-operative of organic farmers in the southeastern part of the state. The landscape was surprisingly beautiful, characterized by dra-

matic bluffs and green rolling valleys. It turned out my new employ-
ers wanted a manager as much as a millwright, but I was eager for
the task. I restored the milling systems and set up national marketing
for their products. Unfortunately, the owner's co-operative ethic did
not extend to the workers that ran to the plant. So, after finishing the
initial work, I left. The plant continued to run for many years until it
finally burned down in the late 80s.

I then had a brief stint in California setting up a system to mill bulk
flour for Erewhon Trading Co. We were primarily blowing the flour
into train cars for pasta production. I was not really happy in L.A.
and missed my beautiful Mississippi River bluff-lands. So I returned
to the Midwest, this time right across the river to Wisconsin, and
founded a small mill and trading company—Little Bear Trading Company. We started with one 16-inch Meadows stone mill and two main
customers. The organic marketplace was growing by leaps and
bounds. Soon our little company was growing at levels of 60-120%
yearly. We introduced the first nationally branded organic tortilla chip,
the first nationally branded organic blue corn chip, the first organic
whole grain croissant, the first healthful natural frosted bran flake
cereal, and our T-shirts with our logo, "Little Bear Flour makes your
bread dance and your cakes sing doo dah" were seen from Paris to
Copenhagen to New York.

My involvement as a manufacturer and as a supplier of organic
grain ingredients has been very rewarding for me in many ways. Over
the years I have been involved in the sale of over ½ billion pounds of
organic processed grain products. I have been involved in the development of organic baby cereals, cold cereals, hot cereals, frozen heat
n' serve croissants, bagels, pizza, entrées of all description, and ingredients from organic food grade alcohol to sweeteners to organic
beer. While president of the national Organic Trade Association
(OFPANA), I was able to take part in the passage of 5 of the 33 state
laws and of the Federal Organic Food Labeling Act. Overall, I feel
that I have been successful in my mission to help bring whole, organic foods to the marketplace.

I am still experiencing the rewards of this mission. I have four
healthy children. When they were young they were not immune from
illness, but they certainly have had less illness then their peers. I attribute much of this to the effects of a balanced diet of primarily organic food products. On a broader level, I have witnessed what can

only be described as a revolution in the eating habits of Americans. The category that was once on the top of the food pyramid (meat) is now on the bottom. Whole grain products are recognized as a very necessary part of any healthful diet. The growth rate of over 20% per year for the last 4 years attests to the viability and broad base of organic food sales.

Why do people buy organic food products? Many appreciate the safe food aspect. There is virtually no danger of synthetic chemical pollution when there is no application to the growing plant and none used in further processing. This is of primary importance to people with many kinds of allergies, as well as to people who are concerned about the long-term health risks posed by chemical applications. Some buy organic foods to support the family farmers that produce organic raw materials. Organic farming can offer a viable response to the giant feed lots and corporate farms that often pollute our rural areas. Some consumers are buying organic foods to aid in cleaning up the environment. If synthetic chemical applications are eliminated, the farm source point pollution is reduced or eliminated. I believe that it is important whenever possible to stress these positive aspects of organic foods.

Over the years, I have been involved in many panel discussions concerning the need for control of the use of pesticides and herbicides in food production. As the organic industry flourishes, I hear the discussion about food shortages and bad quality crops less and less each time. The pesticide company representatives that formerly told me their chemicals did not stay in the soil or the plant because they were water soluble, no longer state this openly due to rising concerns over water quality issues. My position has been one of cautious conservatism. If it is possible to grow and manufacture food without synthetic chemicals, why would anyone want to add unnecessary costs to their already small gross incomes, to say nothing of the health risks involved in applying such substances?

Many organic farmers actually achieve as high or higher yields than conventional farmers do. But organic farming can be a difficult learning process for some growers. To qualify as organically grown, one must grow crops on land that has not had a synthetic chemical application for 36—48 months. The premiums that most organic growers achieve will not be available during this transition period. Also, farmers in this period are learning new approaches to farming that may take them some time to perfect. So, at the onset, yields may potentially go down without the accompanying price increase for certified organically labeled sales. However, prices to growers after that period range from 30%-75% above local market. Organic growers may have lower yields, but they also have lower input costs: they do not have the expense of costly synthetic fertilizers, herbicides, and pesticides. In an elaborate study done by the USDA in the mid 70's, it was concluded that if every farmer in America converted to organic farming the price of food would rise slightly to everyone except organic farmers. The primary losers in this scenario would be the giant agricultural chemical (usually petroleum related) producers.

Although many consumers are familiar with the agricultural chemicals currently used by farmers, many are unaware of the toxicity of the chemicals used in food processing. In milling, compounds are used that, under another label, are considered to be biological warfare components. Is it really possible that there are no traces left of these processing and storage aids in the food we eat? Some of the readers will be old enough to remember the ethylene di-bromide fiasco. This pesticide was discovered in the water that a former governor of California was drinking. This discovery led him to start a hunt for the sources of EDB and it was found to be in use as a fumigant in flour milling. It was finally banned by EPA, and many conventional food companies were forced to recall cake mixes, flour etc. because of their high concentrations of EDB. EDB has now been replaced by phostoxin (Aluminum Phosphide), also known as phosgene gas, exposure to which can be deadly. I am not reassured by this replacement.

The good news is that it is now possible to produce almost any food product using organically grown ingredients and acceptable processing methods and to distribute these food products anywhere and everywhere in the USA. I have taken part in the production of almost every food category sold today in the mainstream supermarkets, as well as in the natural food stores. Major companies such as Proctor & Gamble (Millstone label/organic coffee) and ConAgra, with certified organic production plants, are recognizing the consumer interest in organic food products. H J Heinz, who recently purchased the Earth's Best Organic Baby Food Company, is another large company with a growing investment in the organic movement. The market is expected to be almost 5 billion dollars this year at retail level.

Although this is less than 3% of the total American food market, every percent is enough to waken the conventional food giants who are continually fighting over ever-smaller percentages.

What does the future hold? As many proponents of traditional wisdom have expressed it, we are all interconnected. Every action that we take has some affect on the planet and all those that inhabit this fragile envelope of life that exists on the surface of the earth. We all have the ability to choose. Once we have clearly seen that we are poisoning ourselves and our earth, air, and water, we can only look for a sane and practical methodology to heal and replenish our Ecosphere. To ignore this would be foolish. If the chemicals in our air, water, earth and food are not necessary to promote life, why risk their usage. No one knows the cumulative or synergistic effects of many of the compounds that we still use and consume daily.

So what action can we take? I urge you to look more carefully at the food choices you make. Look for a statement that your food is certified organic. There are several credible organic certification organizations. Part of the Federal Organic Food Labeling Act involves the creation of uniform federal guidelines for organic foods. Look for the organic certification organizations that monitor the organic food processes. It is their job to oversee the production of your food from the seed and grower to the processor and seller. Learn about certification from one of these independent organic certification organizations by calling their offices and asking for promotional materials or seek their website on the Internet. As one of my old clients used to say, "be a label detective."

I cannot live in peace in my little pocket of sanity in southern Wisconsin and ignore the larger issues that affect us all. We are all brothers and sisters. We must work together on viable solutions to create the life supporting and enhancing foods that we desire and need. I can suggest some small steps to take that can make a difference. If you have any room at all, grow some of your own food organically. I think that you will find that the satisfactions and rewards of this activity will extend far beyond just having wholesome, fresh produce to enjoy. When you shop, regardless of where you shop, request certified organic food from your grocer. Whenever possible, buy organic food products. If they cost more, remember that we are losing as many as 20% of our farmers every year. Your purchase is a vote for the preservation of the family farm and sustainable agriculture.

Although I live in rural America, I see here the same move to centralization that we are witnessing in major urban centers. Yet I continue to look forward to a renaissance in our approach to food processing and distribution. I have firmly believed for the last 30 years that the best approach to food production and distribution is through decentralization. Organic farming encourages decentralization. I have given testimony in many state legislatures on the need for local agriculturally related businesses. Although there are many large organic farms, they tend to be smaller than conventional farms and are usually family run operations. I believe that we will all be healthier, as will our environment, if we begin to support localization of food production. We must each demand to know what is "in" our food and endeavor to promote high quality, sustainable organic food products, for our health and the health of our children. Remember in the final analysis, "you *are* what you eat."

When tillage begins other arts follow.
The farmers therefore are the founders
of human civilization.

—DANIEL WEBSTER

How ironic that in this hour of revolution and departure
from the traditional wisdom of our agrarian forefathers
we continue to use the word "farm" whose roots
(ML. *Firma, firmare, firmus*)
imply a more steadfast relationship with the earth.

—EDITOR

Why Organic?
Reversing the Environmental
Impact of Modern Agriculture

EXCERPTED FROM A LECTURE GIVEN BY GENE KAHN, CEO OF CASCADIAN FARMS, AT THE ANAHEIM NATURAL PRODUCTS EXPO, MARCH OF 1995. BY PERMISSION OF CASCADIAN FARMS.

History Of Agriculture

For the first few million years of human life, food needs were met by hunting and gathering. Agriculture began only about 6-8000 years ago. If human time on earth were a 24-hour clock, in which 100,000 years equaled an hour, and human life began at midnight, they lived as hunter-gatherers for nearly the whole day, from midnight thru dawn, to noon, and thru sunset. Finally, at 11:54 PM, agriculture started. Human beings altered their environment from the beginning. Mass extinction of species followed the arrival of human beings on every continent. Hunting and gathering provided what appears to have been a very balanced diet, making tall, strong, healthy individuals. However, the evidence from physical anthropology shows that after agriculture began, health and height decreased, and death from disease and malnutrition increased. This may have been because agriculture allowed for more people, depending on a few staple, carbohydrate crops. Surpluses and population growth created the rise of cities and civilization, but also shortages and malnutrition.

In *Topsoil* and *Civilization*, Carter and Dale show how agriculture began where there was a combination of fertile soil, moisture and flat tillable land. The Nile River Valley, for example, was a place where nature had, for centuries, deposited rich, alluvial soils. Agriculture, from its beginnings, reversed that process. The quality and quantity of soils declined. Writers of history seldom note the importance of land use. They don't mention that conquerors and colonizers had often ruined their own land before they went off to take that of others. The decline of many civilizations resulted from a failure to conserve resources. Most lasted only 1000-1500 years, or 40-60 generations. Some examples are the Minoans of Crete, the Maya of the Yucatan and the Anazazi of our own Southwest. How did early humans destroy or deplete their environment? They cut down or burned all the usable timber, they overgrazed and denuded grass lands. They killed most wildlife and over fished streams, rivers and coast lines. Reservoirs and irrigation systems filled with silt.

Resource Base

One standard formula for human enterprise is: capital + labor + raw materials + management x technology = progress. The equation would usually consider raw materials as a constant, but they aren't constant. Soil fertility, usable waterforce, grass, beneficial wildlife and other resources have not remained a fixed quantity at any time, in any region. They have decreased in most areas occupied by "civilized" man, and have almost disappeared in many of the older countries. They are not the only factor which determines the fate of a civilization, but they are basic limiting factors.

Modern "Industrial" Agriculture

Modern agriculture, as we know it, began in 1842 with Justus von Liebig, who discovered that three basic elements of plant nutrition, Nitrogen, Phosphorus and Potassium, (the "NPK" or "20-20-20" we know from the side of fertilizer bags) could be dissolved in water and fed directly to plants. In combination with innovations in seed hybridization and the mechanization of labor the use of these chemically formulated fertilizers resulted in incredible increases in productivity and population, first in industrialized countries, and subsequently in developing countries. But a short-term burst of plant nutrients, often reduce the long term capacity of the soil to grow crops. They do so by killing off many soil organisms, and rendering the soil more powdery and vulnerable to erosion. Thus, increases in productivity and population throughout our century came at the expense of the resource base. While the use of chemical fertilizers world wide increased, the incremental gain in productivity for each additional ton applied decreased.

What are the natural resources necessary for food production? They are: Soil, moisture, temperature, light, seed, and of course, labor. Take any one element away, and things collapse. Nature has evolved many specific interactions that make up what we call life. In each species of plant and animal some combination of these elements occur. We understand some of the general processes, for example: photosynthesis, respiration, transpiration, germination. As you look at this list you can see that all the elements are related. You can see that for any specific food crop the relationships between elements are very specific, tangible. Oranges only thrive in certain temperatures. Cranberries require so much moisture. Agriculture has always been a relationship of humans with the complexity, and the simplicity of all these processes that go on in plant growth. Sometimes relating with some knowledge and skill, sometimes with ignorance and recklessness. Perhaps one difference between organic agriculture and conventional agriculture is how much awareness and respect we have for what we don't know. This is to say, what we can learn from nature.

So...Out of the interaction of these elements comes food. The equation: Soil Health>leads to>Plant Health>leads to>Food Nutrition>leads to>Human health expresses the interconnectedness of all life through the food chain. It is the cornerstone of Organic Agriculture, as articulated by a number of its founders:

- Sir Albert Howard, working with agriculture in India, demonstrated the necessity of returning nutrients to the soil that have been removed in the process of farming. This was done especially through the use of compost.
- His disciple, Lady Eve Balfour, formed the British Soil Association, to further research and educate on the relationship of healthy soil to human nutrition.
- In the U.S., J.I. and Robert Rodale published Organic Gardening, New Farm, and Prevention magazines, and Paul Keene founded Walnut Acres.
- The Biodynamic Association in Europe and the U.S., following the teachings of Rudolph Steiner, also emphasized the use of compost, and the importance of soil health.

All researched the nutrition in organic/vs/conventional foods. Increasingly there are findings of higher protein, amino acids, vitamin and trace mineral levels in organic foods, all of which are related to immunity and health.

Costs of 'Agribusiness'

In less than a century, while modern agriculture has given us incredible productivity and "cheap food," it has also brought us enormous environmental problems. Rachel Carson in her book *Silent Spring* countered the prevailing optimism of the "Green Revolution," by documenting the early evidence of terrible effects of pesticide usage on wildlife. We have had several decades now since Silent Spring to observe a continuing degradation of the environment. Perhaps because it happens over years, the scope of the damage is still difficult to comprehend. One way is to try to quantify the costs of cleaning up water pollution or soil erosion, or of the social and health services required to replace lost community infrastructures. Some economists take these externalized "costs" which are outside the normal equation by which we figure food costs and prices now, and try to calculate what would happen to our "cheap food" supply if those costs were internalized. That is, if they were figured into the price at the checkstand. Some of the losses are impossible, of course, to quantify. For example, the numbers of lost species, or the loss in quality of life from ill health, can't be measured in dollars. Furthermore, many losses are not only cumulative, but compound, and whole bio-systems collapse when one key element goes.

Report Card

Now let's look at the report card for agriculture's last 60 years. World Resources Institute stated in 1992:

"Global Food Production has increased substantially over the past two decades, but factors such as population pressures and environmental degradation are undermining agriculture's current condition and future prospects."

The resource base, fossil fuels, soils, minerals, genetic and water resources have been drawn to levels that in many cases cannot be replaced.

Soil Erosion

- The United States loses 3.1 billion tons of topsoil annually to erosion.
- About 23% of the U.S.'s cropland loses twice the SCS-established tolerable amount every year. This is 15-30 times faster than soil is formed by nature.
- Off-farm costs of dealing with soil sedimentation have been estimated at between $2-$6 billion annually. Economic loss is estimated at $45-60 billion.

Soil Contamination

Contamination of agricultural soils, particularly by persistent older pesticides like DDT, Dieldrin, Aldicarb, etc., are documented in all major agricultural areas, even twenty or more years after their actual use. Uptake and concentration of soil-residual chemicals by root crops and curcurbits like squash and melons is a problem.

Soil Quality

The loss of Soil Quality from compacting and the loss of organic matter is another consequence of industrial, petroleum-intensive agriculture. Chemical fertilizers and intensive cultivation promote more rapid oxidation of soil organic matter, and tractors cause compacting. Both result in the loss of microbial life in the soil. Continuous cropping in some places, without rotations, has resulted in the loss of as much as 66% of soil organic matter in just 30 year time. Earthworms digest organic matter in healthy soils, depositing tons of fertile castings. Their absence signals soil sterility.

Water Pollution

Nitrates, pesticides, and industrial chemicals are found in both surface and ground water in 46 percent of all counties in the United States. Many commonly-used pesticides are water soluble and are therefore known to leach into groundwater supplies.

Problems from Pesticide Use

In 1985 the American Chemical Society said one billion pounds of synthetic organic pesticides were produced in the U.S., representing about 50,000 products, based on about 1400 active ingredients. Agriculture was estimated to use about 77% of that. This represented a 40—fold increase from 1950. About 90% of all herbicide and pesticide usage is on 4 crops: corn, cotton, soybeans and wheat.

Resistance

Despite this intensive use, in the last forty years the percentage of crop losses from insect damage has doubled, and the percentage of crops lost to disease has increased as well. Pesticide resistance now develops so rapidly, it often appears within just a year or two of introduction. As one Commentator put it, pest resistance to pesticides is like "natural selection in fast forward."

Exposure

Pesticide exposures are, for the most part, cumulative. That is, health damage is not from a single direct exposure, so much as from the additive affects of many low doses over a lifetime. Direct exposures also occur, resulting in a life-long disability known as "Multiple Chemical Sensitivity." Proving correlations or specific cause and effect relationships between a chemical and a health problem is difficult. Multiple exposures over time to many different substances is the rule, and isolating each variable, difficult. Evidence shows that infants and children are susceptible to lower dose exposures than adults. Toxicity testing is normally done on small mammals, and does not usually test for the effects of combinations of substances.

Residue Testing

In figures released by the USDA Pesticide Data Program from a 1992 supermarket-basket survey, the results were startling. While only 63 (about 1%) of the samples had "illegal" residue levels, all but 40% of samples had some detected residues. Apples, peaches and celery had residues in over 80 samples. Multiple residues were found in many samples and in all crops tested.

Health Effects

Pesticides move up the food chain from field crops fed to animals, to livestock products eaten by humans, and there concentrated and stored in fat tissues. While long term effects of pesticide exposures are still largely unknown, health effects have been established. Permanent damage to reproduction, immunity, neurologic function and metabolic systems of both humans and other "non-target" species have been shown to be pesticide related.

These include:

- 50% decrease in sperm counts in American men since 1940
- 5 million women in the US have Endometriosis, which has been linked to dioxin exposures at extremely low levels. (parts per trillion)
- Cancer of the testes tripled in three decades in US and Britain.
- Prostate cancer doubled in the last ten years.
- Abnormal sexual development, thinned egg shells, high infant mortality is found in 40-50% of birds, alligators.
- DDT and DDE are linked to a rise in breast cancer rates, from one women in twenty in 1960, to one in nine in 1994.

Pesticide Regulation Fails To Keep Up

Despite these findings, enforcement of pesticide regulation continues to lag very far behind. A 1989 report from Congress noted that just 2% of 30 billion pounds of imported food was actually tested by the FDA, and of that, 40% failed. Of 300 pesticides which Congress directed the EPA to review in 1972, only 30 have yet had review, and none completely. 15 pesticides identified as "probable carcinogens" have not been withdrawn from use. The "lag time" it takes for unknown affects to become "known" is well-illustrated by DDT:

DDT was introduced in 1942 to help control malaria-causing mosquitoes. The first mosquito resistance to it was noted only 6 years later. Affects on wildlife were noted in the 1950's and '60's. DDT was banned in the U.S. in 1972. It was definitively linked with breast cancer in 1992. With a half life of 59 years in temperate climates, it is still residual in many agricultural soils. It is still being manufactured and used in developing countries.

Other Problems for Modern Agriculture—

Which I can't take time to elaborate on now are: ENERGY, INEFFI-CIENCY, MONOCULTURES & BIODIVERSITY, DWINDLING GLO-BAL WATER SUPPLIES, and their relationship with deforestation and Global Warming, the Loss of Farmland to Development, and the Loss of Farmers. Organic agriculture is challenged to address these problems, as other problems must be addressed: in ways that enhance, rather than deplete, the resource base.

Strategies/Techniques of Organic Agriculture

Organic agriculture's methods are practical, effective and increasingly economically viable as alternatives to conventional methods. Imitating nature's own complex relationships, organic agriculture emphasizes building and maintaining soil fertility, recycling wastes, and establishing a diverse community of plant and insect life.

Soil Building—the use of cover crops and green manure's to increase soil organic matter, nitrogen, and other nutrients in organic agriculture has positive affects on soil structure, microbial activity and thus on plants' ability to take up balanced nutrients, and to resist stress. While chemical fertilizers feed plants while burning up soil, composts and organic matter feed the soil, and thus the plants. Because of the rising cost of petroleum based fertilizers, many farmers have returned to traditional methods of cover-cropping, legume rotations, and the use of animal manure's to maintain fertility In commodity crops this can be very cost effective, because of the lowered input costs.

Composting, from a household scale to a municipal and large farm scale, is the mixing of combinations of organic wastes—plant materials, food scraps, manures, food processing waste, fish, kelps, etc. and their decomposition into humus. Humus is the organic matter that is the basis of fertility. As it is digested by worms and soil microorganisms, nutrients are made available to plants. The use of composts can help control many plant disease, as well, because of beneficial bacteria they provide.

Pest Management Through Diversification and Habitat Creation

To get off the "pesticide treadmill" organic farmers use many different, innovative methods of pest and disease prevention and control. These include regular and frequent field monitoring of pest populations, observing and studying insect behavior and life cycles, and finding ways to work with, or disrupt those cycles. It also involves creating ecosystems within the farm and its borders that provide habitat for beneficial insects and insect-eating birds, alternative feed sources, and "catch crops." Beneficial insects, or bugs that eat other bugs, are all part of the balance, predator and prey, that keeps any one species from getting out of control and becoming a pest. Pesticides can actually make things worse by killing "non-target" insects, including beneficial, thereby upsetting the natural balance. "Bio-controls" utilize specific predator-prey or sexual attraction relationships observed from nature to control insect populations. They include, for example, parasitic bacteria like *bacillus thuringensis*, which when ingested by caterpillars destroys their digestive systems; to sex-pheromone baits which lure coddling moths to traps hung in the apple orchards; or ladybugs which eat many types of aphids which attack many different crops. Limited use is made of plant derived toxicants such as pyrethrin, neem, ryania, etc., for severe infestations.

Integration of Livestock

The integration of livestock in an organic system closes the nutrient loop by returning manures to the soil. Avoiding the toxic accumulations of nitrates in water and diseases which are a problem with intensive conventional livestock systems, rotational grazing and pasture management can supply most feed requirements without purchased inputs and without the erosion of land from over-grazing. Also, many pesticides are used in conventional agriculture on feed crops subsequently fed to animals whose products are eaten by people. This means it is important to build a whole system of clean agriculture; that we eat dairy products, eggs and meats that are raised in systems that do not deplete or pollute natural resources, and are healthy for us.

Weed Control

Many techniques of mechanical cultivation, both old, new and redis-covered, are used in different types of organic cropping systems. Some, like the "weed badger," allow for close cutting of cover crops in be-tween and around perennial vines such as grapes or berries. Others, like "ridge-till" conserve soil and reduce weed germination. Many growers have experimented with "flaming"weeds, early in their growth, before the emergence of the crop seedlings. The use of inter-cropping, cover crops, and perennial permacultures are all strategies for weed control that work with nature's own habit of always cover-ing bare earth with something, and choosing what that will be, in-stead of weeds. Timing is very important in organic weed control, as is the understanding of seasonal succession in weed populations. With an understanding, weeds can also be managed in agricultural sys-tems for the benefits they can bring. For example, weeds "mine" min-eral nutrients from the sub-soil, and act as forage for beneficial in-sects. In some crops the costs of mechanical weeding exceeds costs of herbicides, and results in higher prices for those foods, like carrots.

Social Scale and Integration

Typically, organic farms have been smaller and owner-operated. Mar-keting often is more face-to-face, local or regional, still utilizing natu-ral food distribution channels. Much more than in conventional agri-culture, there are still some real connections between the people on farms who grow the food, people who handle, process and distribute food, and those who buy it. This is what the Japanese mean when they talk about "the face of the farmer." There is a real person behind this food. There are many examples of vertically integrated farm op-erations who process their own crops, and have become for us, names and faces we recognize and trust: Lundbergs, Walnut Acres, Organic Valley.

It must be said, however, that to continue growing, organic food production must continue diversifying in its scale and types of op-erations. At one end we must find economies of scale which allow for the penetration of conventional or mass markets, and at the other end, we must strengthen regional and community farming, where food production can be horizontally integrated into the cultural and social fabric of our daily lives.

To paraphrase Paul Hawken from his book, *The Ecology of Commerce*, "the solutions to cleaning up hazardous wastes do not lie in introducing more novel substances into the environment. Instead the successful technologies of the future will be those that are most efficient in utilizing natural processes and conserving resources.....such as organic farming."

To quote Bernard M. Baruch: "During my 87 years, I have witnessed a whole succession of technological revolution. But none of them has done away with the need for character in the individual or the ability to think." I hope this presentation has given you some food for thought.

They that have the power to hurt and will do none. . .
husband nature's riches from expense.

—SHAKESPEARE

Nature is trying hard to make as succeed,
but nature does not depend on us.
We are not the only experiment.

—BUCKMINSTER FULLER

My best friend,
what do you like?
You said
the corn
is my pleasure.

—SIOUX SONG

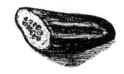

The Evolution of *Organic*

GRACE GERSHUNY, M.S.

The concept of "organic" agriculture has evolved in opposition to the industrial model of food production that became dominant in the latter half of the twentieth century. However, the organic model has always emphasized a positive alternative to the chemical approach to food production. As such, organic practices point the way to a better understanding of the relationship between humans and the earth. We are not simply opposing the destructive qualities of conventional systems, we are creating and describing a more wholistic approach to life. While organic food is often marketed to consumers based on a negative claim about the absence of potentially harmful chemicals, the practice of organic agriculture requires a positive commitment to using sophisticated, ecologically sound management methods.

The organic model is more than just an alternative agricultural technology; it is an integrative world view. The organic world view is also expressed in other areas, such as health, housing, transportation, and even spirituality. This approach is given political prominence today through the increasing emphasis on "sustainable development" as a domestic and international policy goal. First and foremost, the organic world view replaces the notion of domination with one of cooperation. Domination of nature is the premise on which industrial agriculture is based, and which is responsible for the ill effects wrought by modern chemical warfare on weeds, pests, and diseases. Corollary to this is the idea of scarcity–unless we subdue nature, there will not be enough food for everyone. As has been amply demonstrated by authors such as Frances Moore Lappe, however, hunger is the result of inequitable economic systems, which deny the poor access to food and land, not inadequate supplies of food. The tragedy of the industrial model is that it ignores the social and political dimensions of food production and distribution, and thus "requires" environmental degradation as the only recourse to alleviating the suffering of famine, disease and poverty.

Organic agriculture emphasizes cooperation with nature, observation and mimicry of ecological relationships, and maintaining balances. Its practice requires patience, curiosity, open mindedness and humility. Organic farming implies a commitment to non-aggression, and solving problems without casting nature as an adversary. Rather than picking up the sprayer when they encounter an insect problem, organic farmers recognize the pest as a symptom of some imbalance in their system. Knowing that even "natural" pesticides kill predator insects indiscriminately, they will only use these substances as a last resort.

The age of chemical agriculture arrived around the time of Darwin, when a German chemist named Justis Von Liebig proved that plants could take up simple compounds of nitrogen, phosphorus and potassium to convert them to protein and carbohydrates. This discovery did not immediately capture the market but its usage expanded during the aftermath of WWI when the munitions manufacturers were casting about for a market for large stockpiles of nitrate based explosives. Why not sell it to farmers as fertilizer? The new scientific approach to farming had a great deal of appeal, since it was much easier to handle chemicals than haul cartloads of manure to the fields. What's more, these fertilizers really did make plants grow quickly and yield more. But as soon as the artificial manures started becoming popular, a few farmers started to notice that something was amiss. Seeds were losing their vigor, and crops seemed to lack a certain vital quality. They brought their concerns to the renowned Austrian mystic Rudolph Steiner, and he obliged them with a series of lectures that focused on preparing compost and building soil humus to restore the lost vitality to crops. Thus was born the first alternative agriculture movement, which today is known as Biodynamic farming.

As the modern era advanced, agriculture became more and more industrialized, in keeping with the prevailing faith in scientific improvement, efficiency, and specialization. World War II brought new sophistication in chemical warfare, leading to the creation of yet another stockpile of weaponry, this time in the form of insecticides and herbicides, that found a new market in the agricultural sector. The war on nature escalated, with victory holding the promise of universal prosperity undreamed of when farmers were at the mercy of pests, weeds and diseases. The failure of this dream was recognized only by a few skeptics at first. Here and there were voices, such as Edward Hyams, whose warnings about the destruction of precious topsoil were driven home by the clouds of Oklahoma soil that darkened the skies as far away as Washington, D.C. In the forties scientists such as Sir Albert Howard, William Albrecht , and Lady Eve Balfour began demonstrating that proper crop and livestock nutrition depended more than was generally acknowledged on complex, living soil.

There are different claims about who first used the word "organic" to describe the alternative to chemical-intensive agriculture, but without a doubt the greatest popularizer of this concept was J.I. Rodale, who founded the publishing and research organizations that remain among the leading proponents of this approach. The public's awareness of the dangers of chemical-intensive agriculture was aroused in the early sixties by Rachel Carson, giving rise to the modern environmental movement. A "new wave" of organic farming advocates and activists was spawned by the diverse streams of consciousness awakened during this period, including the civil rights and peace movements. With their emphasis on non-violent opposition to injustice, egalitarian decision making, and a utopian vision of a more harmonious social order, the reverse migration of urbanites to rural areas during this era injected a new enthusiasm into the development and spread of ecologically oriented technologies.

The idealism of the sixties and early seventies was tempered by the hard reality of economic survival in the "me decade" of the eighties. Appealing theories of working with nature were balanced with the realization that sustaining a farming venture, no matter how ecologically harmonious, required the ability to produce and market a product for which people would pay. Marketing cooperatives, farmers markets, and more recently, community supported agriculture attracted more attention as organic farmers recognized that the marketing infrastructure was part of the problem facing them in the attempt to replace high volume, centralized, mass market oriented food products with something better. Making a living came to require a mix of enterprises and entrepreneurial skills, in addition to the capacity to master the sophisticated techniques of organic production. Professionalism, including attention to appearance and consumer demands, started to assume greater importance.

As the decade of the nineties arrived, the market for organic products was becoming substantial and highly visible. National level organizing among organic farm and certification groups, such as NOFA (Northeast Organic Farming Association), Oregon Tilth, and CCOF (California Certified Organic Farmers), was starting to take place, along with the dawning of awareness that an organic industry now existed, as represented by the Organic Trade Association. In 1989 a *Sixty Minute* expose of the dangers of Alar, a commonly used growth enhancer, created a huge surge in demand for organic fruits, followed by consumers' realization that the supplies of "organic" products that suddenly appeared overnight could not all be legitimate. This event, dubbed "Alar Sunday" by the organic community, led directly to the development and passage of the Organic Foods Production Act (OFPA) of 1990.

The process that led from passage of the OFPA in 1990 to the first publication of USDA's proposed National Organic Program in December of 1997 was a long and painstaking one. During this time, the organic industry continued its exponential growth, and began to look attractive to larger "mainstream" companies such as Heinz, Welch's, and Smuckers. The fastest growing sector of the organic trade has been processed, packaged convenience foods. The specter of an industrialized organic production system, with many of the economic and social ills of the conventional agribusiness approach, began to appear a real possibility. The decade has also brought increasingly disturbing news on the environment and health front, along with the globalization of trade and the accompanying tightening of corporate control over what we eat, wear, read and think. Mixed into this has been an increased level of public hostility towards any and all government activities, exemplified by the horrendous terrorist attack on federal workers in Oklahoma City.

The groundwork that was laid for the USDA's program was built on the principles of organic agriculture that evolved within the movement itself. The definition and statements of principles that follow were crafted by the National Organic Program staff and reviewed by the National Organic Standards Board, the body established under the OFPA to represent the organic community and provide recommendations about how to implement this program. This document represents a summary of the essential concepts that comprise the organic approach to agriculture:

Prologue: Moving Towards Sustainability

The specific set of rules which delineate organic agricultural systems have evolved out of a wider imperative towards sustainable social, economic and cultural forms. The definition of organic agriculture which follows acknowledges that the goal of sustainability is elusive. However, the extent to which an organic system moves towards sustainability is highlighted as a critical yardstick of its success. In simpler terms, the long-term durability of an organic system is its most important attribute.

Intangible considerations such as personal satisfaction, social responsibility and respect for cultural traditions are inherent to the concept of sustainability. Although beyond the purview of government regulation, they are implicit in organic production systems. In order for an agricultural system to endure, it must be embedded within a social and economic system which equitably rewards all participants, and protects the capability of future generations to feed themselves.

Organic agriculture is a sustainable production management system that promotes and enhances biodiversity, biological cycles and soil biological activity. It is based on minimal use of off-farm inputs and on management practices that restore, maintain and enhance ecological harmony.

"Organic" is a labeling term that denotes products produced in accordance with the standards and certification requirements of the National Organic Program. The principal guidelines for organic production are to use materials and practices that enhance the ecological balance of natural systems and that integrate the parts of the farming system into an ecological whole. Organic agriculture practices cannot ensure that products are completely free of residues. However, methods are used to minimize pollution of air, soil and water. Organic food handlers, processors and retailers adhere to standards to maintain the integrity of organic agriculture products. The primary goal of organic agriculture is to optimize the health and productivity of interdependent communities of soil life, plants, animals and people.

Organic production systems seek to provide food, fiber and herbal products of the highest quality in sufficient quantities. The following principles are the foundation of organic management methods:

1. Protect the environment, minimize pollution, promote health and optimize biological productivity. The primary goal of organic production systems is optimizing environmental health, human health and biological productivity. Organic producers therefore seek to reduce or eliminate reliance on practices and inputs (natural and synthetic) that may harm soil life, deplete nonrenewable resources, pose a hazard to water and air quality, or threaten the health of farm workers or consumers.

2. Replenish and maintain long-term soil fertility by providing optimal conditions for soil biological activity. The health of the soil is fundamental to the health of the whole system, and may be evaluated by the extent and vitality of its biological activity. "Feed the soil, not the plant," continues to be a primary tenet of ecologically sound soil management. Fertility improvement practices must balance physical, chemical and biological considerations to optimize the quantity and diversity of soil organisms. Such practices may include a combination of crop rotations, rotational grazing of livestock, cover crops, intercropping, green manures, recycling of plant and animal wastes, tillage, and judicious application of essential mineral nutrients.

3. Maintain diversity within the farming system and its surroundings and protect and develop plant and wildlife habitat. Biological diversity is a key ecological precept, essential to stability and therefore to sustainability. Diversity must be enhanced in every aspect of organic production, including the selection of inputs, crop varieties, livestock breeds, rotation cycles and pest management strategies. The principle of diversity can be similarly applied to personal skills, social interactions, and economic decisions.

4. Recycle materials and resources to the greatest extent possible within the farm and its surrounding community as part

of a regionally organized agricultural system. Organic producers intensively manage the individual farm system and use biologically-based inputs in preference to petroleum-based inputs. Soil and plant nutrients depleted through cropping and natural leaching are replenished by nutrient sources from within the farm and the surrounding community. Livestock and crop production are integrated wherever possible, to provide the most effective means of nutrient recycling. Energy expended in transportation, manufacturing and handling of agricultural inputs and products is minimized to the greatest extent possible.

5. Provide attentive care that meets both health and behavioral requirements of farm animals. Farm animals are managed to prevent health problems through a focus on diet, housing, handling and observation. Livestock are bred and selected to enhance stamina and vigor. Organically produced feed, in conjunction with care and living conditions which minimize stress, is the foundation of a health promoting management system. Attentive care for the healthy animal is a fundamental precept of organic livestock management.

6. Maintain the integrity and nutritional value of organic food and processed products through each step of the process from planting to consumption. Organically grown food and processed products are processed, manufactured, and handled to preserve their healthful qualities and maintain the principles of the organic management system. Ingredients, additives and processing aids used in organic processed products must be consistent with the overall principles of organic production. Consumers should be provided with the assurance that products bearing organic labels are certified organic by independent verification from seed through sale.

7. Develop and adopt new technologies with consideration for their long range social and ecological impact. New practices, materials and technologies must be evaluated according to established criteria for organic production. It is assumed that organic production systems will continue to progress toward sustainability over time through technical innovation and social evolution.

Each of these seven principles could constitute a book in itself. There is also a key principle that is implied but not stated here. That is, that the term "organically produced" on a product refers to the management system that created the product, including every practice from soil fertility to packaging materials. It does not make any specific claim about product quality. You will note that while the definition speaks of protecting the organic integrity of products there is no claim made that organic products must meet particular product quality standards. Consumers may believe, with some justification, that organic products are better in many ways, and that they are more healthful, but this is a judgment that consumers have to make for themselves after being fully informed about the production methods used. There are also some desirable attributes that may not be offered by an organic label, such as "locally grown." Many consumers prefer to buy produce from the local farm stand, even if small amounts of synthetic chemicals are used, rather than to buy organic produce that has journeyed thousands of miles to reach the supermarket.

When Secretary of Agriculture Dan Glickman announced the publication of the proposed rule on the National Organic Program, he emphasized that the organic label represents a claim about a production process, not product quality, and repeated several times that "this is not about safer food." This proclamation might have been confusing to some consumers who purchase organic food for its health benefits, and there were many responses to the USDA's proposed rule expressing outrage over this statement. In fact, the very same week *Consumer Reports* announced the publication of its findings that organically produced foods were indeed less likely to contain residues of agricultural chemicals than conventional products.

So why did Mr. Glickman make such a statement, if it flies in the face of the reasoning most people use when they choose organic food? The primary reason is that the Secretary of Agriculture could never endorse a program, no matter how beneficial it was, if this were to imply to the public that there is something "wrong" with food produced by conventional agricultural systems. Such an implication would represent a clear affront to the majority of conventional agribusiness interests—an obvious political impossibility. Just as obviously, no one can be expected to embrace a revolutionary change in how they approach their profession and repudiate everything they've been doing for the past fifty years, no matter how open minded they are. But beyond this, there are many important reasons why we are all better served by remembering that an organic label on a product refers to how it is produced, not what it is.

The concept that the *process* is at least as important as the *product* is a revolutionary one, whose importance even many in the organic movement have failed to grasp. The concept allows us to ask the questions that have been ignored, at the peril of society and the planet, by conventional agribusiness. The methods used to produce a product have to be evaluated in terms of their effects on the whole system in which they are used, starting with the soil ecosystem and moving outward to the relationship to water quality, biological diversity, livestock health, and ultimately the nutritional quality of the product. Beyond this, the health of the farm family, the community of which it is a part, and the larger society are all indirect "products" of this process. The quality of the product is one factor in this concept, but rather than being the one and only goal of the production system, a product of high quality becomes a natural outgrowth of a system that is in balance–in a sense, the quality of the product becomes an indicator of the health of the system as a whole. The industrial model emphasizes efficiency of production and counts units produced per acre as the measure of its success. In the organic model, the health of all participants in the production process, from earthworms to watersheds, is the measure of its success.

This world view is the subject of a much larger shift in the world of science and social theory, that is moving beyond reductionist science to holistic, qualitative, and participatory models of arriving at "truth." It is one that may be familiar to chaos theorists and anthropologists as an approach that recognizes multiple possibilities and relationships. Issues are not seen as questions of "either-or," but rather the coexistence of internal contradictions is acknowledged. The possibility of "both and" options changes the very way that choices are made. So, for example, large agribusiness companies can conceivably convert millions of acres of farmland to organic production, destined for processed products such as breakfast burritos, at the same time that activists continue promoting the virtues of buying locally grown foods and joining community supported agriculture farms. The two are not mutually exclusive, and the opportunity to buy organic products in familiar places like supermarkets and even convenience stores may initiate many people, who are unlikely to venture into health food stores, into greater awareness of how their food is produced.

The image of society as a pyramid, with the powerful politicians and corporate chiefs at the top and the poor at the bottom, must change to one of society as an organism composed of many living cells that carry out its various functions in a symbiotic relationship. The margins of society, as described by Wendell Berry in his classic *The Unsettling of America*, are the place of greatest creativity and possibility, the carriers of new ideas and change. In order for these changes to be assimilated by the center of society, the margins must move from the outside in. Social hierarchies and domination of one group by another, mirrored in the notion that humanity must dominate nature to survive, must give way to structures that are neither "top-down" nor "bottom up," but that turn the current social system "inside out."

The concepts and principles discussed here imply that organic agriculture is one step towards a sustainable culture, and that the larger social questions of equity and justice must be also be satisfied in achieving that goal. It is also a goal that we know will constantly recede as we approach it. Nevertheless, it is imperative that we work as diligently as we can to at least move in that direction. The obstacles are enormous, and include our own resistance to change.

Today, as the century that has seen an unprecedented assault by human 'civilization' on its environment draws to a close, the fundamental question facing the organic community is this: Will the organic approach to agriculture be allowed fulfill its potential to replace industrialized agriculture as the most widely practiced mode of production? Can the world view associated with organic agriculture, including an emphasis on cooperation, non-aggression, decentralized economies, and egalitarian values, among others, become accepted along with the shift to a more ecologically sound form of agriculture? For this to happen, the antagonism felt by the organic community towards government, heightened by years of official hostility and resistance to organic methods, will have to be released. Unless "the establishment" is permitted to fully embrace organic principles in agriculture and see for themselves how effective and sensible this approach is, this larger goal will fall short. Organic products will remain the province of the upscale consumer in boutique niche markets and offer no serious alternative to mass-produced industrial food for the majority of people. In order for the young organic concept to mature, its parents must release it from their control and allow it to take its place in the world.

As organic production moves into the mainstream, the government can and should take over the policing role that has, until now, been assumed by (and in some cases, consumed) the organic community. This does not mean that organic advocates can walk away from involvement with the process–there is no escaping the need to continue to collaborate with and carefully scrutinize the public institutions that purport to represent us. However, letting go of full responsibility for enforcing the rules, which of course *must* be compatible with the organic principles discussed here, will free up the energies of the movement to develop and refine the social and ethical implications contained within the organic approach. We can then dare to envision organic agriculture as becoming the new 'conventional' model in the twenty-first century–in fact, the life of the planet demands it.

The choice, after all, is ours to make.
If, having endured much, we have at last asserted
our "right to know," and if, knowing, we have concluded
that we are being asked to take senseless and frightening risks,
then we should no longer accept the counsel of those who tell us
that we must fill our world with poisonous chemical;
we should look about and see what other course is open to us.

—RACHEL CARSON

Deep in the man sits fast his fate
To mould his fortunes mean or great.

—EMERSON

A Final Survey

Sir Albert Howard

THE capital of the nations which is real, permanent, and independent of everything except a market for the products of farming, is the soil. To utilize and also to safeguard this important possession the maintenance of fertility is essential.

In the consideration of soil fertility many things besides agriculture proper are involved—finance, industry, public health, the efficiency of the population, and the future of civilization. In this book, an attempt has been made to deal with the soil in its wider aspects, while devoting due attention to the technical side of the subject.

The Industrial Revolution, by creating a new hunger—that of the machine—and a vast increase in the urban population, has encroached seriously on the world's store of fertility. A rapid transfer of the soil's capital is taking place. This expansion in manufacture and in population would have made little or no difference had the waste products of the factory and the town been faithfully returned to the land. But this has not been done. Instead, the first principle of agriculture has been disregarded: growth has been speeded up, but nothing has been done to accelerate decay. Farming has become unbalanced. The gap between the two halves of the wheel of life has been left unbridged, or it has been filled by a substitute in the shape of artificial manures. The soils of the world are either being worn out and left in ruins, or are being slowly poisoned. All over the world our capital is being squandered. The restoration and maintenance of soil fertility has become a universal problem.

The outward and visible sign of the destruction of soil is the speed at which the menace of soil erosion is growing. The transfer of capital, in the shape of soil fertility, to the profit and loss account of agriculture is being followed by the bankruptcy of the land. The only way this destructive process can be arrested is by restoring the fertility of each field of the catchment area of the rivers which are afflicted by this disease of civilization. This formidable task is going to put some of our oversea administrations to a very severe test.

The slow poisoning of the life of the soil by artificial manures is one of the greatest calamities which has befallen agriculture and mankind. The responsibility for this disaster must be shared equally by the disciples of Liebig and by the economic system under which we are living. The experiments of the Broadbalk field showed that increased crops could be obtained by the skillful use of chemicals. Industry at once manufactured these manures and organized their sale.

The flooding of the English market with cheap food, grown anywhere and anyhow, forced the farmers of this country to throw to the winds the old and well-tried principles of mixed farming, and to save themselves from bankruptcy by reducing the cost of production. But this temporary salvation was paid for by loss of fertility. Mother earth has recorded her disapproval by the steady growth of disease in crops, animals, and mankind. The spraying machine was called in to protect the plant; vaccines and serums the animal; in the last resort the afflicted live stock are slaughtered and burnt. This policy is failing before our eyes. The population, fed on improperly grown food, has to be bolstered up by an expensive system of patent medicines, panel doctors, dispensaries, hospitals, and convalescent homes. A C3 population is being created.

The situation can only be saved by the community as a whole. The first step is to convince it of the danger and to show the road out of this impasse. The connection which exists between a fertile soil and healthy crops, healthy animals and, last but not least, healthy human beings must be made known far and wide. As many resident communities as possible, with sufficient land of their own to produce their vegetables, fruit, milk and milk products, cereals, and meat, must be persuaded to feed themselves and to demonstrate the results of fresh food raised on fertile soil. An important item in education, both in the home and in the school, must be the knowledge of the superiority in taste, quality, and keeping power of food, like vegetables and fruit, grown with humus, over produce raised on artificial. The women of England—the mothers of the generations of the future—will then exert their influence in food reform. Foodstuffs will have to be graded, marketed, and retailed according to the way the soil is manured. The urban communities (which has suffered from exploitation) in making possible the restitution to the country-side of its manurial rights. All connected with the soil—owners, farmers, and laborers—must be assisted financially to restore the lost fertility. Steps must then be taken to safeguard the land of the Empire from the operations of finance. This is essential because our greatest possession is ourselves and because a prosperous and contented country-side is the strongest possible support for the safeguarding of the country's future. Failure to work out a compromise between the needs of the people and of finance can only end in the ruin of both. The mistakes of ancient Rome must be avoided.

One of the agencies which can assist the land to come into its own is agricultural research. A new type of investigator is needed. The research work of the future must be placed in the hands of a few men and women, who have been brought up on the land, who have received a first-class scientific education, and who have inherited a special aptitude for practical farming. They must combine in each one of them practice and science. Travel must be included in their training because a country like Great Britain, for instance, for reasons of climate and geology, cannot provide examples of the dramatic way in which the growth factors operate.

The approach to the problems of farming must be made from the field, not from the laboratory. The discovery of the things that matter is three-quarters of the battle. In this the observant farmer and laborer, who have spent their lives in close contact with Nature, can be of the greatest help to the investigator. The views of the peasantry in all countries are worthy of respect, there is always good reason for their practices, in matters like the cultivation of mixed crops they themselves are still the pioneers. Association with the farmer and the laborer will help research to abandon all false notions of prestige, all ideas of bolstering up their position by methods far too reminiscent of the esoteric priesthoods of the past. All engaged on the land must be brother cultivators together, the investigator of the future will only differ from the farmer in the possession of an extra implement—science—and in the wider experience which travel confers. The future standing of the research worker will depend on success: on ability to show how good farming can be made still better. The illusion that the agricultural community will not adopt improvements will disappear, once the improver can write his message on the land itself instead of in the transactions of the learned societies. The natural leaders of the country-side, as has been abundantly proved in rural India, are only too ready to assist in this work as soon as they are provided with real results. No special organization, for bringing the results of the experiment stations to the farmer, is necessary.

The administration of agricultural research must be reformed. The vast, top-heavy, complicated, and expensive structure, which has grown up by accretion in the British Empire, must be swept away. The time-consuming and ineffective committee must be abolished. The vast volume of print must be curtailed. The expenditure must be reduced. The dictum of Carrel that ' the best way to increase the intelligence of scientists would be to reduce their number' must be implemented. The research applied to agriculture must be of the very best. The men and women who are capable of conducting it need no assistance from the administration beyond the means for their work and protection from interference. One of the chief duties of the Government will be to prevent the research workers themselves from creating an organization which will act as a bar to progress.

The base line of the investigations of the future must be fertile soil. The land must be got into good heart to begin with. The response of the crop and the animal to improved soil conditions must be carefully observed. These are our greatest and most profound experts. We must watch them at work, we must pose to them simple questions, we must build up a case on their replies in ways similar to those Charles Darwin used in his study of the earthworm. Other equally important agencies in research are the insects, fungi, and other micro-organisms which attack the plant and the animal. These are Nature's censors for indicating bad farming. Today the policy is to destroy these priceless agencies and to perpetuate the inefficient crops and animals they are doing their best to remove. Tomorrow we shall regard them as Nature's professors of agriculture and as an essential factor in any rational system of farming. Another valuable method of testing our practice is to observe the effect of time on the variety. If it shows a tendency to run out, something is wrong. If it seems to be permanent, our methods are correct. The efficiency of the agriculture of the future will therefore be measured by the reduction in the number of plant breeders. A few only will be needed when soils become fertile and remain so.

Nature has provided in the forest an example which can be safely copied in transforming wastes into humus—the key to prosperity. This is the basis of the Indore Process. Mixed vegetable and animal wastes can be converted into humus by fungi and bacteria in ninety days, provided they are supplied with water, sufficient air, and a base for neutralizing excessive acidity. As the compost heap is alive, it needs just as much care and attention as the live stock on the farm; otherwise humus of the best quality will not be obtained.

The first step in the manufacture of humus, in countries like Great Britain, is to reform the manure heap—the weakest link in Western agriculture. It is biologically unbalanced because the micro-organisms are deprived of two things needed to make humus—cellulose and sufficient air. It is chemically unstable because it cannot hold itself together—valuable nitrogen and ammonia are being lost to the atmosphere. The urban centres can help agriculture, and incidentally themselves, by providing the farmers with pulverized town wastes for diluting their manure heaps and by releasing it for agriculture and horticulture, the vast volumes of humus lying idle in the controlled tips.

The utilization of humus by the crop depends partly on the mycorrhizal association—the living fungous bridge which connects soil and sap. Nature has gone to great pains to perfect the work of the green leaf by the previous digestion of carbohydrates and proteins. We must make the fullest use of this machinery by keeping up the humus content of the soil. When this is done, quality and health appear in the crop and in the live stock.

Evidence is accumulating that such healthy produce is an important factor in the well-being of mankind. That our own health is not satisfactory is indicated by one example. Carrel states that in the United States alone no less than £700,000,000 a year is spent in medical care. This sum does not include the loss of efficiency resulting from illness. If the restitution of the manurial rights of the soils of the United States can avoid even a quarter of this heavy burden, its importance to the community and to the future of the American people needs no argument. The prophet is always at the mercy of events; nevertheless, I venture to conclude this book with the forecast that at least half the illnesses of mankind will disappear once our food supplies are raised from fertile soil and consumed in a fresh condition.

Who sows a field, or trains a flower,
or plants a tree, is more than all.

—John Greenleaf Whittier

Hurt not the earth,
neither the sea,
nor the trees.

—Revelations 7:3

May it be mine beside Demeter's altar
to dig the great winnowing fan through
her heaps of corn, while she stands smilingly
with sheaves and poppies in her hand.

—A Reaper's Prayer

When the world has the Way,
ambling horses are retired
to fertilize fields.

—Lao Tzu

Postscript: The *Health* in Organic Food Products

DAVID RICHARD

"Organic Coffee Creamer!" my friend incredulously repeated, as if that one phrase might raise J.I. Rodale from his grave and rouse him to overturn the moneychangers' tables within the Organic Food Movement. My friend's wife and I, eating a casual lunch on either side of him during a recent natural food convention, could only join him in shaking our heads. Each of us had witnessed the latest round of organic products to be introduced into the marketplace with some amazement, leading us to wonder what organic product might be introduced next—refined sugar, "enriched" white bread, aerosol deodorant or even cotton candy? As the saying goes—what is missing from this picture?

I sense the futility of these kinds of "innovations" on at least two levels. On a primary level, it seems absurd to invest the amount of biological "capital" and personal "interest" in the soil required by organic agriculture in order to create products whose nutritional value is negligible and whose cumulative effect on health is likely to be negative.

On a more subtle level, it seems down-right dishonest to call a product "organic" when its processing has rendered it less than healthy and whole. After all, the human body is its own ecological system. As Robert Rodale has stated (see page 3), "*Organic* food is not [or should not be] debased by unnecessary processing." [Emphasis added.]

I suggest that those who are developing and marketing organic products need to review their own definition of the term "organic" and build for themselves a philosophical foundation on the concept that "organic" is more than a marketing perspective or even a growing technique: it is an affirmation of life. Unless the health and well-being of the consumers of these products is foremost in the minds of their developers and marketers, the products themselves are unlikely to promote health or well-being. And isn't this what organic products in the food chain really about?

Let's keep things simple and whole in terms of our personal ecology as well as the global ecology. And let's consider each other (and ourselves!) as friends whose health we care about when we introduce a new organic food product or choose to purchase and consume one.

Biographies

Michael Abelman

Michael Abelman has been farming 12 acres of land in the heart of Goleta, California for the last 17 years. He is the founder and director of the Center for Urban Agriculture at Fairview Gardens, a non-profit community education center and national model for urban agriculture which has recently completed a successful campaign to preserve the farm's land from the threat of development. Michael is an internationally acclaimed photographer and author of *From the Good Earth: A Celebration of Growing Food Around the World* (Abrams, 1993) and *On Good Land: The Autobiography of an Urban Farm* (Chronicle Books, 1998).

Dr. William Albrecht

In the 1950's, Dr. William A. Albrecht, Chairman of the Department of Soils at the University of Missouri investigated and promoted soil sustainability in agriculture. His studies linked optimal soil fertility and animal health to organic methods. He also found animals preferred organically grown foods. It was an unprecedented viewpoint at the time given scientific and governmental fascination with agrichemicals and monoculture. These studies became the basis for his book *Soil Fertility and Animal Health*.

Britt Bailey

Britt Bailey is a research associate at The Center for Ethics and Toxics. She has been studying the effects of intensive agricultural practices, particularly biotechnology, upon health and the environment. A surfer and organic gardener, she is an avid supporter of the organic industry. She believes that only *sustainable* agriculture gives back to the environment, better protects farm workers, and provides safe and nutritious food for consumers. Britt is the co-author of a forthcoming book on the genetic engineering of food crops, *Against the Grain: The Genetic Gamble in Agriculture*.

Lady Eve Balfour

Lady Eve Balfour was born in 1898 to a wealthy aristocratic English family. In her early years, she displayed talents as a trombonist and pilot but she is

181

best remembered for her leadership in the organic movement. Her book *Living Soil* (1943) gained world-wide acclaim and led to the formation of the Soil Association of England in 1946. Lady Balfour fittingly served as its first president and was affectionately known as "Mother Earth"—the original title of the Society's magazine.

Christopher Bird

See reference under Tompkins.

Dorie Byers

Dorie Byers' husband says that she has so many farming ancestors that she is drawn to work the soil. This may be true, for she is never happier than when she is planning and planting her gardens. The writings of Rachel Carson and the Rodales inspired Dorie to garden organically outside her home in South Central Indiana. The result is a bountiful harvest of vegetables, herbs, and flowers that she and her family use. Her commitment to organic foods also extends to teaching and writing about organic gardening.

Leslie Cerier

Like many organic food proponents, Leslie "bubbles over" with enthusiasm and energy. An organic chef, caterer, lecturer, teacher and writer, Leslie is busy with several new projects including a couple of books and a new cable TV show which she will host on the Television Food Network. Leslie's first cookbook, *The Quick and Easy Organic Gourmet*, was published in 1996 by Station Hill Openings. In addition to her cooking activities and daily practice of yoga, Leslie finds time to be both a mom and a wife and to cook for friends in her New England home.

Jerry Combs

Jerry is a Professor of Nutrition in the Division of Nutritional Sciences at Cornell University. He teaches courses on "The Vitamins" and "Linking Agriculture and Human Nutrition Needs" and directs a research program focused on issues of micronutrient nutrition. He is internationally known for his work on selenium, his group having found that high intakes of that element can substantially reduce cancer rates. Jerry speaks Chinese and French in addition to his native English and enjoys working overseas. At home, he is active in community theatre.

Trish Crapo

Trish Crapo is a writer who lives on Dancing Bear Farm, a 24-acre organic farm in Leyden, Massachusetts run by her husband, Tom Ashley. She excels at riding the mechanical transplanter, but often finds herself in front of a computer instead. Trish enjoys writing poems and is currently completing a novel.

John Duxbury

John chairs the Department of Soil, Crop and Atmospheric Sciences at Cornell University. A soil chemist by training, John has broad experience in soil management and cropping systems and is a recognized expert on the rice-wheat system of the Indo-Gangetic plains where he directs a project seeking to increase the production of the underlying nutrient system which feeds one-fifth of the world. A soccer fan, John was born in England and raised there, in Zimbabwe and in Rhodesia. He has lived in the U.S. for the past 26 years.

Frank Ford

Born into a farm agents' family during a sandstorm which covered the Texas panhandle in 1933, Frank grew up to become one of the earliest organic farmers in the country and the founder and former president (1960-1996) of Arrowhead Mills. Frank's work ethic, developed through his many childhood jobs and chores and through his training and experience as a nuclear commander in the army, have informed both his personal and professional life. In addition to his professional achievements, Frank spearheaded efforts to prevent the installation of Mx missiles and a nuclear waste dump in farm-rich Deaf Smith Country. Now "retired," Franks energies have been focused on plowing "fields of the spirit" as a volunteer for Campus Crusade for Christ in Asia.

Grace Gershuny

Grace has worked for over twenty years as an organizer, educator and consultant in the alternative agriculture movement as well as being a small-scale market gardener. She is the author of several books and articles on soil management and composting, including *The Soul of the Soil*, coauthored with Joe Smillie, and *Start with the Soil*, published by Rodale Press. Grace was also the editor of *Organic Farmer: The Digest of Sustainable Agriculture* for its four year existence. She has served many roles in the Northeast Organic Farming Association (NOFA) and was a founding member of the Organic Trade Association. Grace has both helped to develop the USDA's National Organic Program and been instrumental in its implementation. She has taught agricultural issues at the Institute for Social Ecology in Plainfield, Vermont for many years and currently serves on the Social Ecology Program faculty at Goddard College. She lives with her husband, Bentley Morgan, and daughter, Opal Hoyt, in Vermont where she grows her own vegetables and is learning about flowers.

Wendy Gordon

Wendy Gordon is the executive director of Mothers and Others for a Livable Planet, a New York based consumer organization she co-founded with Meryl Streep in 1989. Mothers and Others is working to bring about a shift in over-all consumption patterns by focusing on choices that are *healthy, safe* and *environmentally sound*. A wife and mother of two sons, Wendy believes that "environmental change begins in the home." She graduated from Princeton University in 1979 and earned a Masters Degree in Environment Health Sciences from Harvard University in 1982. She has authored or co-authored numerous articles and book chapters related to food, health and the environment, including her own book, *The Groundwater Handbook*, and a forthcoming book concerning the Alar campaign.

Sir Albert Howard

Sir Albert Howard is widely regarded as the founder of the modern organic method of agriculture. He believed that plants should be strengthened in their growth by methods as close to nature as possible. At the turn of the century, he was performing agricultural work in the West Indies and Great Britain when he was appointed Imperial Economic Botanist to the Government of India. While working there, he found that crops were grown nearly pest and disease free by returning plant and animal matter to the soil. He therefor set up an experiment farm and initiated these methods. The culmination of his work is documented in *An Agricultural Testament*, a work that was used as a reference by J.I. Rodale.

Stan Jorstad

The cover photographer, Stan Jorstad, has many stories to tell from his WWII experience in a ski patrol unit stationed in the Italian Alps, from his work with Marlon Perkins as the photographer for the Wild Kingdom television program and from his travels to photograph all fifty-four of our national parks. Stan's book of photographs documenting the beauty of our national park system, *These Rare Lands*, was released in November by Simon and Shuster. Former poet laureate Mark Strand wrote the text for Stan's book and environmentalist Robert Redford contributed the introduction.

Gene Kahn

Gene Kahn is a native Chicagoan who renounced city life in the early 1970's to become an organic farmer in the pristine environment of the upper Skagit Valley in Washington State. From his simple farming activities, surrounded by the beauty of the Cascadian Mountain range, grew the organic farming and manufacturing organization known as Cascadian Farms. Gene's goals are two-fold: to re-focus farmers' attention on the necessity of building permanent, self-sustaining agricultural systems and to encourage consumers to support these systems by purchasing high-quality organic products.

Frederick Kirschenmann

Frederick Kirschenmann was born and raised on the Kirshenmann Family Farms in North Dakota. After earning a doctorate in philosophy from the University of Chicago in 1964, Fred became a teacher, an administrator, and, finally, the academic dean at Curry College in Boston. In 1976, he returned to his family's 3100 acre farm and converted it to sustainable organic production. Fred both helped found Farm Verified Organic, a private certification agency, and now serves as its president. He is currently also a member of the National Organic Standards Board. Fred has published numerous articles and book chapters on sustainable agriculture, and his farm operation and philosophy have been documented in an award-winning video entitled "My Father's Garden."

Dr. Marc Lappé

Dr. Marc Lappé directs a not-for-profit organization, The Center for Ethics and Toxics, where he writes and teaches about the cumulative effects of current technological and agricultural practices. A long-time critic of the overuse of pesticides, he applies his knowledge of history, health policy, toxicology and ethics in his writing. His hope is for a brighter future where health and well-being are not compromised in the name of progress. Marc is the co-author of a forthcoming book on the genetic engineering of food crops, *Against the Grain: The Genetic Gamble in Agriculture.*

Dana Pratt

The winner of the *Taste Life!* essay contest, Dana is a homemaker and homeschool mother of two boys. She has a Master's Degree in Historic Preservation Planning from the University of Illinois at Champaign-Urbana. Dana is an avid Bible student and loves gardening and healthy eating. She lives on a small farm in Central Illinois.

Bargyla Rateaver

Bargyla Rateaver received her Masters and Doctorate Degrees in Botany from the University of Michigan in Ann Arbor, and her master's degree in Library Science from The University of California in Berkeley. A healthy octogenarian, Dr. Rateaver founded the organic movement in California by teaching the first university credit course in the organic method. Her textbook, *The Organic Method Primer*, which she co-authored with her son in 1973, has recently been updated and condensed. For over forty years, Bargyla has dedicated herself to understanding the organic wonders of plants and soil. She hopes to continue to be of service in passing along this understanding.

David Richard

David Richard has been involved in the natural food movement since he worked as a stock boy in his family's health food store as a nine year old "with a big hat" so that customers could see him behind the counter. Over thirty years later, he has managed two health food stores and a brokerage company as well as sourcing natural products from around the world. David is the author of five books, including three on natural health, and two of poetry, and is an enthusiastic consumer of organic products.

J. I. Rodale

J. I. Rodale (1898-1971) was the outspoken publisher, researcher and leader of the organic food movement in the United States. Through his publishing endeavors with Rodale Press which he founded in 1942 and his many books, including the international best seller *Pay Dirt!* (1943), J. I. popularized and expanded upon the philosophy of Sir Albert Howard and brought our country to a new level of understanding of the relationship between the soil and public health. His *Organic Farming and Gardening* (today *Organic Gardening and New Land*) and *Prevention* magazines continue to inform and educate millions in neglected areas of organic practice and natural health. Rodale Press has grown from its humble beginnings to become the largest publisher of health-related books and magazines in the country.

In support of his research, J. I. purchased a 60 acre farm in 1940 which he used to improve and refine his ideas concerning organic agriculture. Today, the Rodale farm at Emmaus, PA serves as a model for sustainable, organic practices.

The legacy of J. I. Rodale continues in his writings, his farm, his publishing business, his research institute and in the millions of people whose lives he influenced.

Robert Rodale

The son of J. I. Rodale, Robert Rodale (1930-1990) was a prolific and persuasive writer and a dynamic leader of the organic food movement in his own right. The author of numerous books and articles including *Save Three Lives— A Plan For Famine Prevention, Living in a Mad World* and *The New Farmer,* Robert served as the Chairman of the Board and Chief Executive officer of Rodale Press for nearly twenty years after the death of his father in 1971. Under his guidance, the company expanded into a broad range of health and fitness related magazines and books supported by four book clubs and a not-for-profit research institute. He also expanded the research farm J. I. founded into a state-of-the-art 305 acre organic agricultural center. An expert skeet shooter and avid bicyclist, Mr. Rodale competed with the U.S. skeet shooting team in the 1968 Olympics in Mexico City.

P. Marc Schwartz

Marc Schwartz is busy working as a consultant with his company, Organic Developments, which serves the organic sector of the natural food industry. Past president of the National Organic Trade Association and current chair of the Organic Grower's and Buyer's Association, Marc traces his roots in the organic movement to the founding of the OGBA with the Rodales in Pennsylvania with whom he was well acquainted. Highlighting his numerous experiences developing organic products, Marc was the founder and first CEO of Little Bear Trading Company. Marc lives in an earth-sheltered, solar-heated home which he built in a wilderness area of Wisconsin. He still grows about half of his own food using organic methods, and both of his daughters have grown up to manage organic food companies.

Peter Tomkins

Mr. Tompkins is an eclectic writer, biographer and historian. In addition to *The Secret Life of Plants,* he has co-authored *Secrets of the Soil: New Age Solutions for Restoring our Planet* with Christopher Bird. He has also written books on the Great Pyramid of Cheops in Egypt, the pyramids of the ancient Central American cultures, *A Spy in Rome, The Murder of Admiral Darlan* and several other works. His most recent book (1997) is *The Secret Life of Nature: Living in Harmony With the Hidden World of Nature Spirits from Fairies to Quarks.*

Ross Welch

Ross is a scientist at the U.S. Plant, Soil and Nutrition Laboratory located on the Cornell University Campus. This USDA laboratory is the only research facility in the world explicitly commissioned to address problems in the food system through interdisciplinary approaches. Ross, an internationally known plant nutritionist, is also a leader of Cornell's Food Systems for Improved Health Program. Outside of his research, Ross is an accomplished woodworker, specializing in crafting fine furniture.

References

From Soil to Plant to Plate

[1] Rateaver, B. & Rateaver, G. (1993) Organic Method Primer UPDATE. San Diego: Rateavers.

[2] R. Linderman. Mycorrhizosphere, (1997) (personal communication).

[3] J.N. Ladd. 1985. Soil Enzymes, in D. Vaughn & R.E. Malcolm, Soil Organic Matter & Biological Activity. Boston. Nijhoff/Dr. W. Junk.

[4] Jackson, W.R. Humic, Fulvic and Microbial Balance: Organic Soils Conditioning. 1993. Evergreen, CO. Jackson Research Center.

[5] Kononova, M.M. 1966. Soil Organic Matter. Elmsford, NY: Pergamon 1. Rateaver, B. & Rateaver, G. (1993) Organic Method Primer UPDATE. San Diego: Rateavers.

Why I Consume Organic Food

[1] Robert C. Oelhaf, Organic Agriculture (New York, Allanheld, Osmun & Co., 1978), pp. 8-9.

[2] Harold E. Butram, M.D. and Richard Piccola, M.H.A., Our Toxic World: Who is Looking After Our Children?, (Quakertown, PA, Healing Research Center, 1997), Ch. 2.

[3] The Staff of Organic Gardening and Farming, The Basic Book of Organically Grown Foods, ed. by M.C. Goldman and William H. Hylton (Emmaus, PA, Rodale Press Inc., 1972) p. 10.

[4] Ibid., p. 11.

[5] Ibid., p. 11.

[6] Justin Wiser, "Organics: Acting Locally," Earth Times, (San Diego, Sept., 1996), p. 1.

[7] Delia Hitz, "Local Organic Foods Markets: Healthy and Growing," Earth Times, (San Diego, Sept., 1995), p.p. 3-4.

[8] Oelhaf, p. 227.

Organic Agriculture and the World Food Supply

[1] A more extensive version of this paper was published in J. Patrick Madden and Scott G. Chaplowe, For all Generations World Agriculture More Sustainable, 1997. World Sustainable Agriculture Publication.

Baskin, Yvonne. 1996. "Curbing Undesirable Invaders." *BioScience*, Vol. 46, No.10.

Bagla, Pallava and Jocelyn Kaiser. 1996. "India's Spreading Health Crisis Draws Global Arsenic Experts." *Science*. (Vol. 274, October 11)

Clancy, Sharon et. al. 1993. *Farming Practices for a Sustainable Agriculture in North Dakota*. Carrington, North Dakota: Carrington Research and Extension Center Report.

Easterbrook, Gregg. 1996. "Forgotten Benefactor of Humanity." *The Atlantic Monthly*. (January)

Flora, Cornelia Butler. 1996. "The Sustainable Agriculturist and the New Economy." Minnesota Department of Agriculture: Energy and Sustainable Agriculture Program.

Food 2000—Global Policies for Sustainable Agriculture, Report to the World Commission on Environment and Development. 1987. Zed Books.

Fox, Nicols. 1997. *Spoiled: The Dangerous Truth About A Food Chain Gone Haywire*. New York: Basic Books.

Hewitt, Tracy I. and Katherine R. Smith. 1995. "Intensive Agriculture and Environmental Quality: Examining the Newest Agricultural Myth." Greenbelt, Maryland: Henry A. Wallace Institute for Alternative Agriculture Report.

Kirschenmann, Frederick. 1997. "Expanding the Vision of Sustainable Agriculture." in Patrick Madden (ed.) *For All Generations*. World Sustainable Agriculture Association

Kloppenburg, Jack Jr. et. al. 1996. "Coming Into the Foodshed." *Agriculture and Human Values*. (Vol. 13, No. 3)

Lappe, Francis Moore and Joseph Collins. 1986. *World Hunger: Twelve Myths*. New York: Grove Press.

National Research Council. 1996. *Lost Crops of Africa: Volume I, Grains*. Washington, D.C.: National Academy Press.

Norberg-Hodge, Helena. 1991. *Ancient Futures: Learning From Ladakh*. San Francisco: Sierra Club Books.

Rifkin, Jeremy. 1992. Beyond Beef: The Rise and Fall of the Cattle Culture. New York: Dutton.

Rissler, Jane and Margaret Mellon. 1996. *The Ecological Risks of Engineered Crops*. Cambridge: The MIT Press.

Schneider, Stephen H. 1976. *The Genesis Strategy: Climate and Global Survival*. New York: Plenum Press.

Shiva, Vandana. 1991. *The Violence of the Green Revolution*. London: Zed Books Ltd.

Snow, Allison A., and Pedro Moran Palma. 1997. "Commercialization of Transgenic Plants: Potential Ecological Risks." *BioScience*. (Vol. 47, No. 2. February)

Soule, Judy. et. al. 1990. "Ecological Impact of Modern Agriculture." in C. R. Carroll et. al. (ed.) *Agroecology*. New York: McGraw Hill.

Spindler, Audrey A. and Janice D. Schultz. 1996. "Comparison of Dietary Variety and Ethnic Food Consumption among Chinese, Chinese-American and White American Women. *Agriculture and Human Values.* (Vol. 13. No. 3).

My Husband's Clover Plants: or, *Why We Farm Organically*

* Organic Farming Research Foundation, P.O. Box 440, Santa Cruz, CA 95061; 408-426-6606 (ph); 408-426-6670 (fax); research@OFRF.org (e-mail).

† The Human Face of Sustainable Agriculture: Adding People to the Environmental Agenda, by Patricia Allen; Center for Agroecology and Sustainable Food Systems, University of California, Santa Cruz, CA .

§ A Time to Act: A Report of the USDA National Commission on Small Farms, January 1998; Miscellaneous Publication 1545 (MP-1545). This report contains many statistics pertinent to small farms, and makes recommendations to the USDA which link the viability of small family farms to "sustainable agriculture" practices. It can be downloaded from the Internet from the following site: http://www.reeusda.gov/agsys/smallfarm/ncosf.htm.

Sustainable Food System Approaches to Improving Nutrition and Health-Nutrition and Agricultural Science.

[1] Division of Nutritional Sciences, Cornell University, Ithaca, NY 14853, USA (corresponding author).

[2] U.S. Plant, Soil and Nutrition Laboratory, USDA, Cornell University, Ithaca, NY 14853, USA

[3] Department of Soil, Crop and Atmospheric Sciences, Cornell University, Ithaca, NY 14853, USA

Barefield, E. 1996. Osteoporosis-related hip fractures cost $13 billion to $18 billion yearly. FoodReview (January-April):31-36.

Brown, L.R. 1995. Who Will Feed China? W.W. Norton & Co., New York and London.

Brown, L.R. 1996. Tough Choices: Facing the Challenge of Food Scarcity. W.W. Norton & Co., New York and London.

Combs, G.F., Jr., R.M. Welch, J.M. Duxbury, N.T. Uphoff, and M.C. Nesheim (eds). 1996. Food-Based Approaches to Preventing Micronutrient Malnutrition: An International Research Agenda. Cornell University, Ithaca, New York.

Frazão, E. The American diet: A costly health problem. 1996. FoodReview (January-April):2-6

Graham, R.D., and R.M. Welch. 1996. Breeding for staple food crops with high micronutrient density. Agriculture Strategies for Micronutrients Working Paper 3. International Food Policy Research Institute, Washington, D.C.

House, W.A., D.R. Van Campen, and R.M. Welch. 1996. Influence of dietary sulfur-containing amino acids on the bioavailability to rats of zinc in corn kernels. Nutrition Research 16:225-235.

House, W.A., D.R. Van Campen, and R.M. Welch. 1997. Dietary methionine status and its relation to the bioavailability to rats of zinc in corn kernels with varying methionine content. Nutrition Research 17:65-76.

Kantor, L.S. 1996. Many Americans are not meeting food guide pyramid dietary recommendations. FoodReview (January-April):7-15.

PHNFLAASH. 1995. Sri Lanka's poverty alleviation project: A review of the food supplement Thriposha. The World Bank Human Development Department. Electronic Newsletter on Population, Health, and Nutrition Issues. Issue 85, August 30.

Ross, E.B. 1996. Malthusianism and agricultural development: False premises, false promises. Biotechnology and Development Monitor 26:24.

UNACC-SN. 1992a. Overview. In Second Report on the World Nutrition Situation, Vol. I. Global and Regional Results. United Nations Administrative Committee on Coordination, Subcommittee on Nutrition. World Health Organization, Geneva. Chapter 1, pp. 4-16.

UNACC-SN. 1992b. Regional Trends in Nutrition. In Second Report on the World Nutrition Situation, Vol. I. Global and Regional Results. United Nations Administrative Committee on Coordination, Subcommittee on Nutrition. World Health Organization, Geneva. Chapter 2, pp. 17-38.

UNACC-SN. 1993. Micronutrient Deficiency: The Global Situation. United Nations Administrative Committee on Coordination, Subcommittee on Nutrition. SCN News 9:11-16.

UN-FAO. 1997. FAOSTAT Agricultural Data. United Nations Food and Agricultural Organization. http://apps,fao.org/cgi-bin/nph-db.pl?subset=agriculture.

USDA-ARS. 1996. Mutant corn has low phytic acid. Agricultural Research 44:12-14. Agricultural Research Service, U.S. Dept. of Agriculture, Washington, D.C.

Uvin, P. 1994. The state of world hunger. Nutrition Reviews 52:151-161.

Welch, R.M. 1993. Zinc concentration and forms in plants for humans and animals. In A.D. Robson (ed). Zinc in Soils and Plants. Proceedings of the International Symposium on Zinc in Soils and Plants, University of Western Australia, 27-28 September, 1993. Kluwer Academic Publishers, London. pp. 183-195.

Organic Foods and Pesticide Use

1. Chuck Benbrook, et al., *Pest Management at the Crossroads*. (Yonkers, NY: Consumer Union, 1996).

2. Theo Colborn, Dianne Dumanoski and John Peterson Myers, *Our Stolen Future: Are We Threatening Our Fertility, Intelligence, and Survival? A Scientific Detective Story* (NY: Plume/Penguin, 1997).

3. Anne Garland, *The Way We Grow*. (New York: Berkley Books, 1993).

4. Joan Gussow, *Chicken Little, Tomato Sauce & Agriculture*. (New York: The Bootstrap Press, 1991).

5. Joan Dye Gussow and Katherine L. Clancy, "Dietary Guidelines for Sustainability," *Journal of Nutrition Education*, Vol.18, No.1, 1986.

6. National Research Council. *Pesticides in the Diets of Infants and Children.* Mothers & Others, 1997, *The Green Food Shopper: An Activist's Guide to Changing the Food System* (New York).

7. Mothers & Others, 1995, "Eight Simple Steps to A New Green Diet: How to Shop for the Earth, Cook for Your Health and Bring Pleasure Back into Your Kitchen" (New York).

8. National Research Council, *Alternative Agriculture.* (Washington, DC: National Academy Press, 1989).

9. National Research Council, *Pesticides in the Diet of Infants and Children.* (Washington, DC: National Academy Press, 1993).

10. Natural Resources Defense Council, *Putting Children First: Making Pesticide Levels in Food Safer for Infants & Children.* (New York: Natural Resources Defense Council, 1998).

Beyond the Romance: Human and Ecological Values of Organic Farming

1. Baker, Beth, *"Harmful algal blooms." BioScience* 48.1 (1997) 12.

2. National Research Council, *Pesticides on the Diets of Infants and Children* (Washington D.C.: National Academy Press, 1993).

3. "Greener Greens: The Truth about Organic Food." *Consumer Reports* Jan. 1992: 14.

4. Potashnik, G., A. Porath, "Dibromochloropropane (DBCP): A 17 year assessment of testicular function and reproductive performance," *Journal of Occupational and Environmental Medicine* 37.11 (1995): 1287-1292.

5. Washington (National Academy Press) 1993.

6. Acuna, MC, V. Diaz, R. Tapia, M.A. comsille, "Assessment of neurotoxic effects of methyl bromide in exposed workers," *Rev. Med. Chil.* 125.1 (1997): 36-42.

7. Liebman, James, *Rising Tide* (San Francisco: CPR, 1997).

8. Hussein, Mian Akbar, "Consequences and Impact of High External Input-Based Agriculture and NGO's Efforts." Organic World (Barra, Dhaka) 1995.

9. Vandameer, John. "Biodiversity Loss in and Around Agroecosystems." Biodiversity and Human Health Eds. Grifo, Francesac and Rosenthal, J. Island Press (Washington, D.C.) 1997: 111-128.

10. Abdel-Mallek, A.Y., M.I.A. Abdel-Kader, and A.M.A. Shonkeir, "Effect of glyphosate on fungal population, respiration and the decay of some organic matters in Egyptian soil." Microbial. Res. 149. (1994): 69-73.

11. Wilson, E.O. The Diversity of Life. Norton (New York). 1992

The Evolution of Organic

Berry, Wendell. *The Unsettling of America: Culture and Agricuture.* Sierra Club Books, 1977. Chapter 9, "Margins."

"Organic Food: Greener Greens?" in *Consumer Reports*, Vol. 63, No. 1, January 1988, pp. 12-18.